Walter Künzel (Editor)

Geriatric Dentistry in Eastern European Countries

Geriatric Dentistry

in Eastern European Countries

Editor

Walter Künzel
Professor Dr. sc. med.

Erfurt

Quintessence Publishing Co., Inc.
Chicago, London, Berlin, São Paulo, Tokyo
and Hong Kong

Library of Congress Cataloging-in-Publication Data

Geriatric dentistry in Eastern European countries / editor, Walter Künzel.
p. cm.
Includes bibliographical references.
Includes index.
ISBN 0-86715-223-0
1. Aged – Dental care – Europe, Eastern – Congresses,
I. Künzel, Walter.
[DNLM: 1. Geriatric Dentristry – Europe, Eastern. WU 490 G3695]
RK55.A3G48 1991
362.1'989776'00947 – dc20
DNLM/DLC
for Library of Congress 90-9095
CIP

Lithography: JUP, Industrie- und Presseklischee GmbH, Berlin
Composition: VPA, Landshut
Printing: Felgentreff & Goebel, Berlin
Binding: Heinz Stein, Berlin

Table of Contents

Contributors List

Baschanow, N.N., Prof. Dr.,
Chair of Stomatology, I. Medical Institute, Moscow, USSR

Borutta, Annerose, Asst. Prof. Dr.sc.med.,
Department of Preventive Dentistry, Faculty of Stomatology, Medical Academy of Erfurt

Dapecí, Alena, Asst. Prof., MUDr.
Second Stomatology Clinic, Medical Faculty, J.E. Purkyne University, Brno, Czechoslovakia

Heinrich, Roswitha, Dr.sc.med.,
Department of Preventive Dentistry, Faculty of Stomatology, Medical Academy of Erfurt

Höcker, M., Asst. Prof. Dr.sc.med.,
Faculty of Stomatology (Charité), Humboldt University, Berlin

Jolov, Z., Dr.med.,
Ministry of Health, Sofia, Bulgaria

Lenz, E., Prof. Dr.sc.med.,
Department of Prosthetic Dentistry, Faculty of Stomatology, Medical Academy of Erfurt

Mareš, V., Asst. Prof. MUDr.
Faculty Hospital, Charles University, Prague, Czechoslovakia

Mari, A., Prof. Dr.med.,
Dental and Maxillofacial Surgery Clinics Albert Szent-Györgyi Medical University, Szeged, Hungary

Rode, M., Asst. Prof. Dr.sc.
Medical Faculty, University of Ljubljana, Yugoslavia

Šicha, V., Prof.MUDr. CSc.,
Institut for Continuing Education of Paramedical Personnel, Brno, Czechoslovakia

Vrbic, V., Prof.Dr.sc.,
Medical Faculty, University of Ljubljana, Yugoslavia

Preface

I envy nothing, I let it pass,
and many things leave me entirely cold;
But to see rows of young teeth without envy, alas
that is the greatest trial of my old age.

None less than Johann Wolfgang von Goethe has thus expressed vividly the yearning of the elderly for preservation of their own teeth.

The apparently inevitable “edentulousness” of the aged, virtually a certainty in the past, at least until the beginning of this century, is being overcome step by step. Ever more often, people retain their own natural teeth longer, even to advanced old age. This is one result of developing, and frequently more effective, dental care, but also the result of increasingly widespread oral health consciousness. The scientifically based concept of lifelong retention of the natural teeth is thus slowly becoming an epidemiologically demonstrable reality in the population; this changing trend must find specific support. Nevertheless, the oral health of the aging population, particularly in those over age 65, is not always satisfactory. Many explanations can be advanced for this; not least the reducing demand of the aged for dental care, and its limited availability. Closing this gap in the health care system requires the formulation of scientifically well founded strategies to improve dental care. These must take existing demographic, infrastructural, economic and personnel conditions into account.

A symposium of experts was held in Brno, Czechoslovakia, in May, 1986, to discuss these problems. Specific topics were addressed by experts from the East European Countries (People's Republic of Bulgaria, Czechoslovakia, German Democratic Republic (GDR), Poland, the Union of Soviet Socialist Republics and Yugoslavia). Following extensive discussions, "Recommendations for further development of dental care of older and aged persons" were formulated. That document provides an orientation of health policy goals and duties of dentists, and the possibilities for organizational changes in provision of geriatric dental care. Although the concept proposed must be fitted in the first instance to the structural requirements of a governmental care system, the Recommendations offer numerous starting points for improvements in care and improved methods for geriatric dental tasks. The International Quintessence Group therefore deserves thanks for agreeing to publish the keynote addresses and for its "recommendation" that thees be made available in English, German and Russian, to make them accessible to a wide range of interested persons. May the conceptionally condensed concepts lead to improved dental care for the elderly of many nations.

Walter Künzel

Part I Introduction

Chapter 1
Conceptual Demands of Oral Health Care for the Elderly

W. Künzel, Erfurt

The elderly and the aged have always been of central interest to dentistry. Convincing evidence of this is the existence of prosthodontics as a special discipline within dentistry. Nonetheless, the more recent international literature contains numerous publications that depict dental care of the aged as a new priority [27, 35]. There may be many reasons for this. Developing theoretical and clinical understanding of the oral cavity environment and its destruction by disease, taken together with advances in technique and materials science, afford new possibilities in diagnosis, treatment and rehabilitation, all requiring adaptation to benefit the patient. On the other hand, a measurable improvement in oral health and the changing age structure of the population is shaking the conventional concept of care[6], requiring reorganization of its aims. It can be assumed that very effective oral health care delivery systems with high accessibility are available in the industrialized nations of the world, in which superbly trained dentists, auxiliaries and dental technicians ensure quality dental care generally acceptable to the population. Multinational comparisons of effectiveness among variously structured oral health care systems [3, 33] have made it clear, however, that the apparently curative and rehabilitative aims of care need redirection to a preventive orientation so that the prerequisites for gradual improvements in oral health status, leading to life-long maintenance of the natural teeth, can be achieved. This process is generation – dependent and assumes age – related priorities in the preventive care of various population groups.

Laws and ministerial decrees regulate dental care in the eastern European nations. In particular, they prescribe the systematic coverage of specific target groups. These include pregnant women and young mothers, children and adolescents (in an organized paediatric dental care system), and a not insignificant number of adults who undergo periodic dental check-ups through industrial health programmes. The result of complex preventive measures is readily seen in the growing number of young people whose oral health status is better than that of earlier generations. It is becoming increasingly clear that the problems of dental care in defined population groups will be solved in the foreseeable future. This will make it possible to redeploy some of the dental potential to other population groups.

As a result, it was not without scientific and health policy foundations that the IXth Conference of Presidents and General Secretaries of the dental societies of the eastern European nations, meeting in Lublin, Poland in 1984, selected geriatric dentistry as the central topic of the 1986 Xth Conference, which was held in Erfurt, GDR. The discussion at that time indicated that dental care of the aged was becoming increasingly important in most countries. This is the consequence in part, of social progress and in part, of demographic changes. To that extent, provision of dental care to the elderly and to aged population groups has a new quality, the meaning and dimensions of which remain to be determined.

Definition of geriatric dentistry

"Whilst geriatric dentistry is the term recommended by the National Library of Medicine, and is widely used in the English language it is, in our view, not necessarily the best term".

Aging, according to *Bürger*[12], is defined as "every irreversible change of living substance as a function of time" (biomorphosis). It includes alterations of material, functional and psychological processes that characterize the individual from its conception to its natural death. As the science of aging of living organisms, including man, it was defined as "gerontology" by *Rybnikow*[42]. The human life cycle is a closed process with loosely defined, meshed phases. Senescence is initiated through a "break" in the efficiency curve, usually around age 45 years, and can lead to senility at age 65. The WHO differentiates between:

aging (45 to 59 years)
elderly (60 to 74 years)
old (75 years =) and
very old (from age 90 years).

Needless to say, the chronological age gradually deviates from biological age.

Although the terms "elderly" and "old", or "seniors" are used below, the life span beyond age 60 years is meant, independently of both biological or health status and of degree of active participation in an occupation or retirement.

Geriatrics[38], also discribed as clinical gerontology, is the branch of medicine dealing with aging in man. Its special concern is the aetiology and the course of diseases in aging and aged persons, and their prevention, diagnosis, and treatment[18]. Although this was the terminological basis for geriatric dentistry, as defined by *Franks* and *Hedegard* [19], *Massler* [37], and *Holm-Pedersen* and *Loe* [24], it does not describe the totality of the biological, nosological and social demands made specifically of dental care in the elderly and the aged. Quite properly, from the point of view of health policy, gerohygiene, i.e. social gerontology, is perceived as a part of gerontology. It may be defined as "the aging- and age-dependent change in psychophysical and social health, depending on relations to and changes in the environment"[15]. *Wilke*[51] attempted to account for the dentally relevant portion of this idea with the term "gerostomatohygiene", but as yet no generally accepted agreement about appropriate terminology exists for the more clearly developing contours of dentistry for the aged.

Some possible trends appeared for the first time in 1983 with the successful founding of the International Association of Gerodontology (IAG); this appears to be a move in the direction of replacing such terms as geriodontology[21,55], gerodontostomatology [9], geriodontostomatology [2], gerontostomatology [39,43], stomatogerontology and stomatogeriatrics [4] and oral gerontology [34] as well as "gerodontology"[45]. Other concepts, such as geroprosthetics [30], orofacial gerontosurgery [14] and prosthetic gerontostomatology [54] describe only specific partial aspects. At least since *Balogh*[4], the word gerostomatology [17] has become more widely accepted. Continuation of the use of the term is found in *Breustedt*[10,11] and *Antalovska*[1]; these Hungarian authors intended that the term should indicate the scientific basis of dental care for the aged as a discipline of dentistry, rather than the reverse, i.e. as a subspeciality of geriatric medicine. Logically, the concept includes communal determination of social and medical care of the aging and the aged patient, also integrating oral care [46].

Aging of populations

Since the turn of the century, the proportion of aging and elderly has tripled [25]. This is a part of the "long life revolution" that is still continuing. Thus, for example, the International Association of Gerontology, in its petition to the World Conference of the United Nations, noted that the century

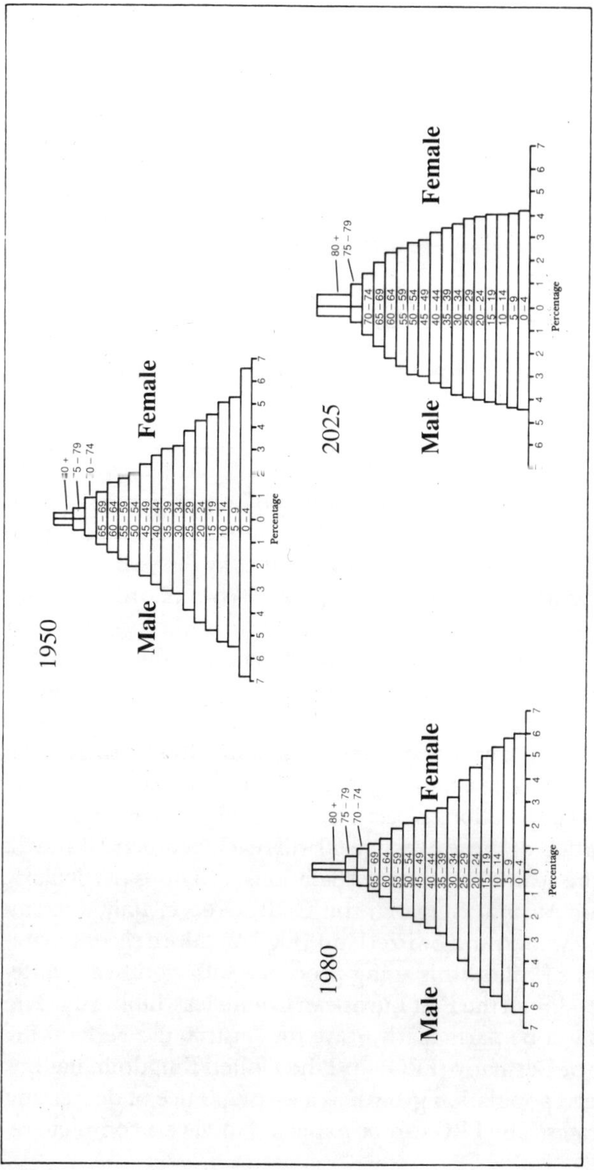

Fig. 1-1 Age-sex pyramid of the world population in 1950, 1980 and 2025.

Table 1-1 Estimated Percentage of population aged 65 and more in selected countries [48].

Country	1990	1995	2000	2010	2020	2025
Cuba	8.2	8.6	8.9	10.9	12.7	13.3
Korea	3.8	4.0	4.4	5.2	6.7	8.3
Vietnam	4.1	4.2	4.3	4.7	5.5	7.1
Bulgaria	12.7	14.0	15.1	15.1	16.4	16.7
Czechoslovakia	11.6	12.1	12.2	12.5	15.6	16.2
GDR	12.7	12.9	13.7	16.3	16.8	18.0
Hungary	13.5	14.4	14.9	15.5	18.3	19.0
Poland	10.0	11.1	12.0	11.9	15.3	17.1
Rumania	10.2	11.4	12.5	12.8	13.8	14.5
Yugoslavia	9.2	10.9	12.6	13.7	16.1	17.3
USSR	9.4	11.1	11.9	12.5	13.3	14.8

of youth has changed into a century of senior citizens [44]. The proportion of the population living into old age is constantly increasing; it may be anticipated that by the year 2000, the 1980 figure for those over age 60, 376 million, will have doubled, and that by the year 2025, this will have led to a world-wide alteration in the age structure of the population (Fig 1-1). Taking a global view, there is a fear that this aging of the population will lead to increasing pension costs (public and private), stagnation, possible loss of societal vitality and, not least, intergenerational conflicts [13].

Aging of populations is particularly significant in Europe. The proportion of those over age 60 will reach between 18 and 22 % by the year 2000 in 19 of 28 nations [52]. This is particularly true for Austria, Bulgaria, the GDR, Greece, Italy, Luxembourg, Sweden and Switzerland (Fig 1-2). More recent extrapolations [48] show this aging process – with significant differences – for all the East European Countries (Table 1-1). The effects will be particularly grave for Austria, the Federal Republic of Germany (FRG) and the United Kingdom, nations with zero population growth as a consequence of decreasing birth rates. The FRG can be expected to have a complete reversal of its age structure by the year 2030 (Fig 1-3), by comparison with the actual data from 1910 (Germany) and 1975. It may be assumed that every seventh person in Europe in the year 2025 will be over 60 years old. In such a population structure, the age groups with a high need for social and medical care increase proportionally, a matter that also has relevance to dental care strategies.

Oral health status and degree of care

Drafting prospective care strategies requires precise, demandoriented formulation of parameters that measure health indictors accurately and reproducibly. These must be sufficiently sensitive and sufficiently specific to mirror changes in the epidemiological situation [6]. From the dental point of view, (1) clinically perceptible caries amenable to treatment, and (2) functional natural teeth meet this requirement. While the caries rate is a particularly good comparative indicator of oral health in children and adolescents, the existence of functional natural teeth – or edentulousness as the final result of the disease process – serves the same function in adults and the elderly. Demonstration of natural teeth in the oral cavity, without attempting to determine their functional usefulness, has been developed internationally as a measure of the general health of a population [16], analogously to infant and child mortality.

While a great deal of information exists about the prevalence of caries and gingivitis in the adolescent population (national and WHO data banks), knowledge about the prevalence of oral disease and the extent of dental care of middle-aged and elderly adults is limited.

The best international comparison is provided by the ICS-I (International Collaborative Study of Dental Manpower Systems) data [3]. One result of this study is that 13- and 14-year-old children of the participating nations can be classi-

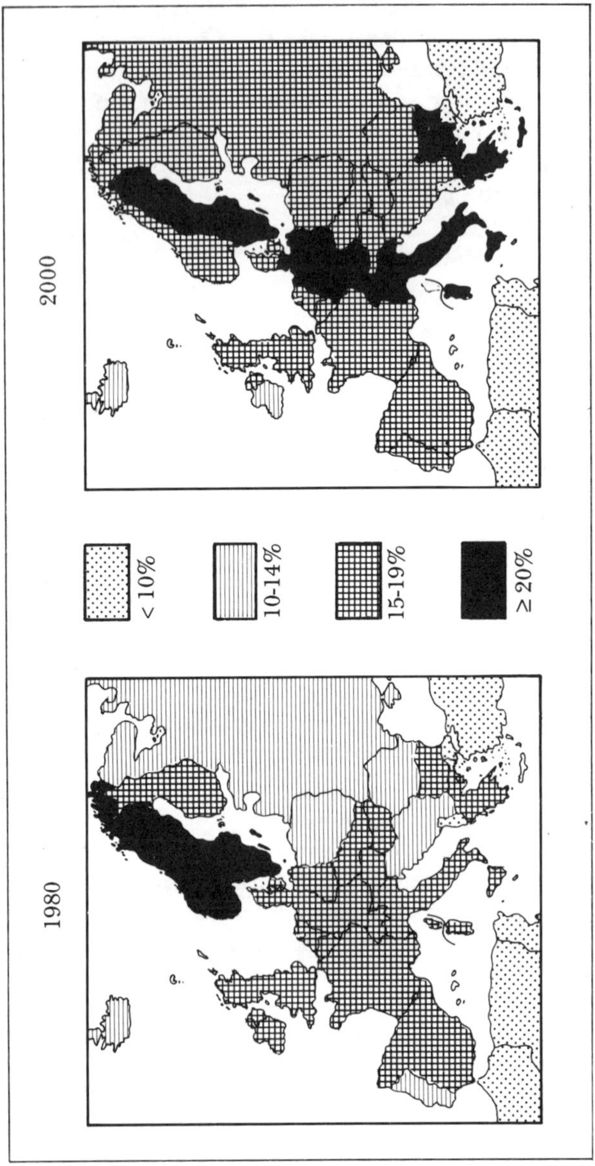

Fig. 1-2 Population trends in the European Region; estimated percentage of population aged 60 years and over (United Nations, 1979).

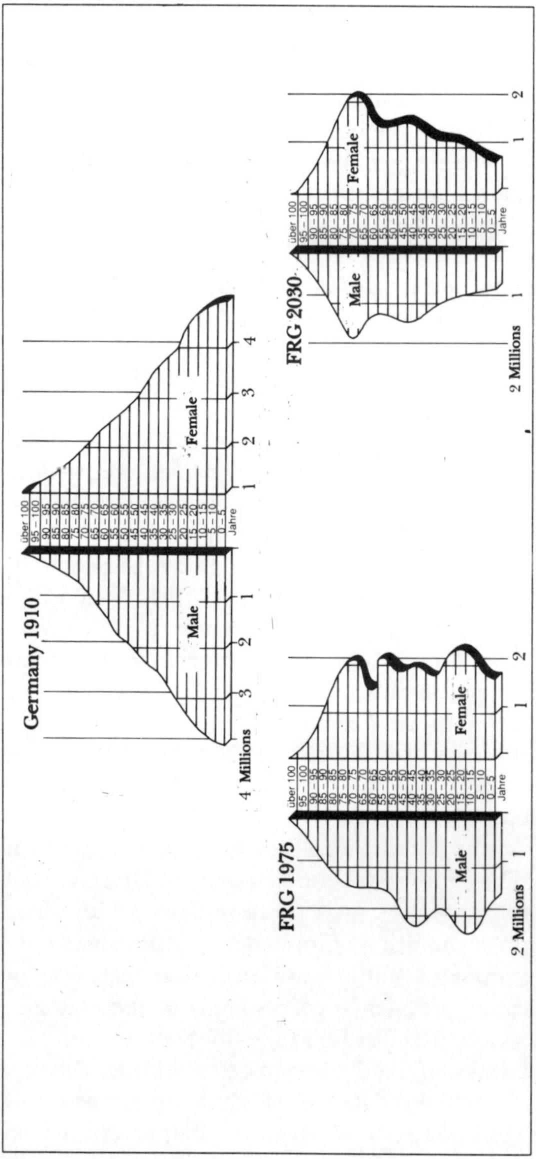

Fig. 1-3 Age pyramid of population in the Federal Republic of Germany in 1975 compared to the situation in Germany in 1910 and the estimated number of inhabitants by the year 2000; left = male, right = female. Changes of typical age pyramid in consequence of "zero-growth" an aging of populations.

fied into low, medium and high caries prevalence groups (Fig 1-4), and that this classification persists to the age category 35 to 44 years (Fig 1-5). For example, prevalence in the GDR is low and in Poland it is high. This is reflected in the number of demonstrable natural teeth per individual, and finally in the percentage of edentulousness (Fig 1-6). While the rate of edentulousness is between 8% and 36% in such nations as Australia, New Zealand and the United States, it does not exceed 1% in the GDR [29,53].

This depicts the most important epidemiological priority for better oral health among senior citizens, even if it would require a relatively extensive amount of prosthetic care and restoration. Randomized test samplings in the GDR regions of Erfurt and Leipzig [7], and in Karl-Marx-Stadt [49] document a generally acceptable prosthetic status (Fig 1-7), as indicated by the proportion of persons having fixed and removable prostheses. The number with prostheses increases to a greater epidemiological proportion only after age 60 [8].

Edentulousness among those over age 65 is reported as 8% in 1973 in Ireland, 58.7% in Norway in 1975, 55.9% in Australia in 1984, and 82.6% in The Netherlands in 1977 (WHO data bank, 1988). In the GDR, the proportion of edentulous persons over age 65 varies between 20% and 80% [22].

This generation of senior citizens, with limited dental function in a series of industrialized nations of the world, stands in contrast to a young generation which, because of caries preventive measures, is characterized by improved oral health status and drastically reduced needs for treatment [20, 40]. The caries reduction rate of up to 70% is accompanied by a 30% to 50% increase in probands with caries-free dentition, a condition of immediate significance to the general development of the dentition [32]. The secular trend change in caries prevalence corresponds to the changing pattern of periodontal disease in the population. Here, it is not so much a matter of reduction in prevalence as of change in severity. Increasingly, less serious disease forms occur, more easily controllable through secondary preventive mea-

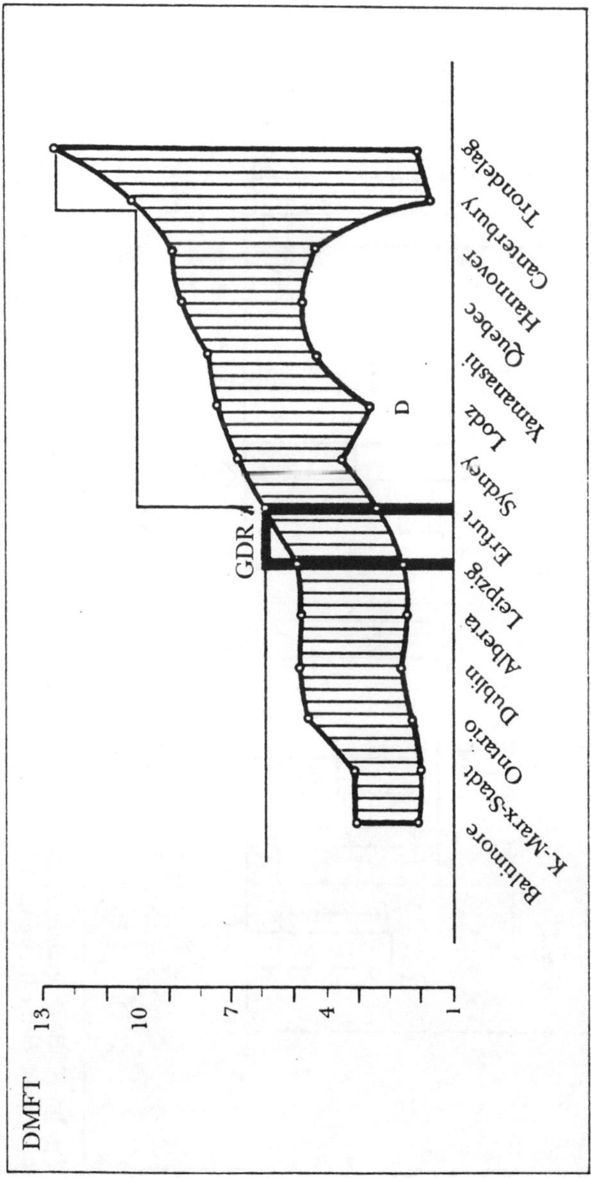

Fig. 1-4 Caries prevalence (FM and D) in the age group 13 to 14 in study areas of the International Collaborative Study of Dental Manpower Systems (WHO, 1985).

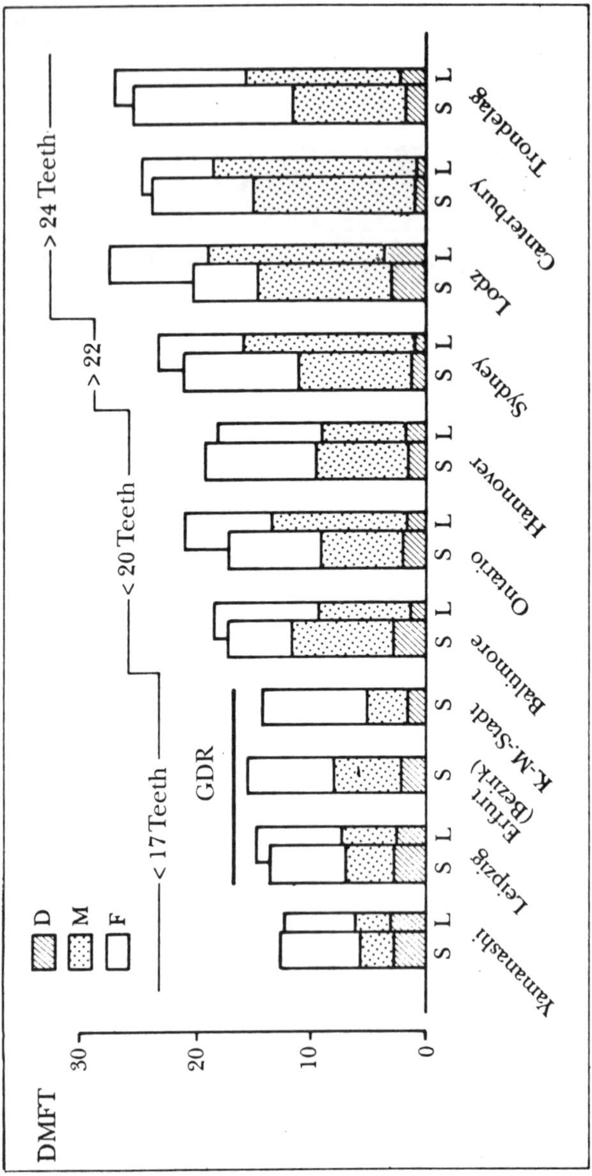

Fig. 1-5 Caries prevalence and mean number of filled, missing and natural teeth in the age group 35 to 44 in study areas of the International Collaborative Study of Dental Manpower Systems (*Borutta* et al., 1988).

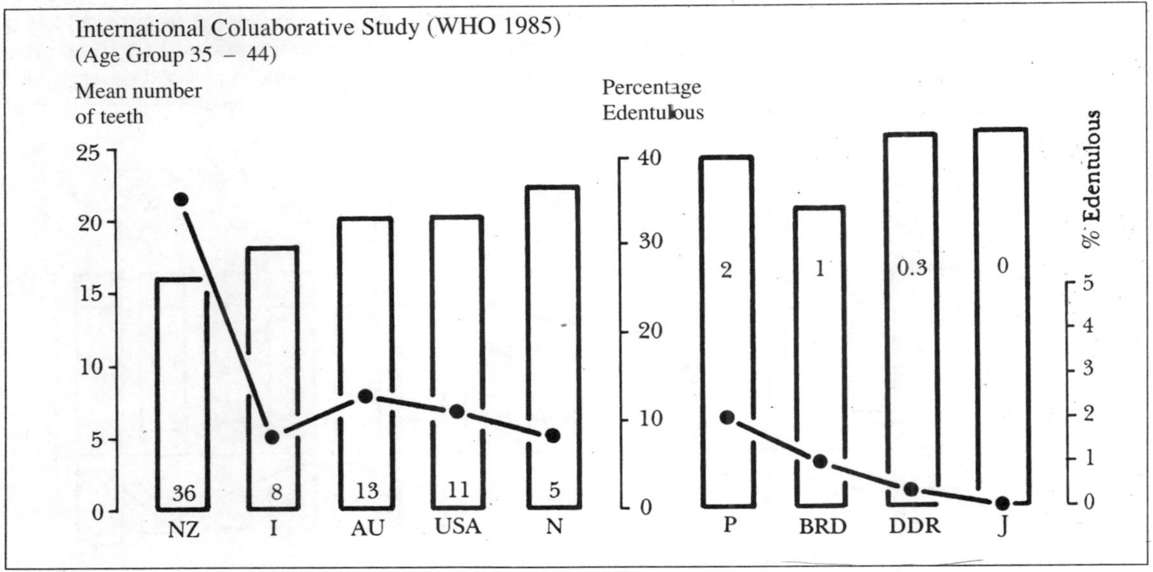

Fig. 1-6 Number of natural teeth and percentage of edentulous (age-group 35 to 44) in study areas of the International Collaborative Study of Dental Manpower Systems (WHO, 1985); country names abbreviated

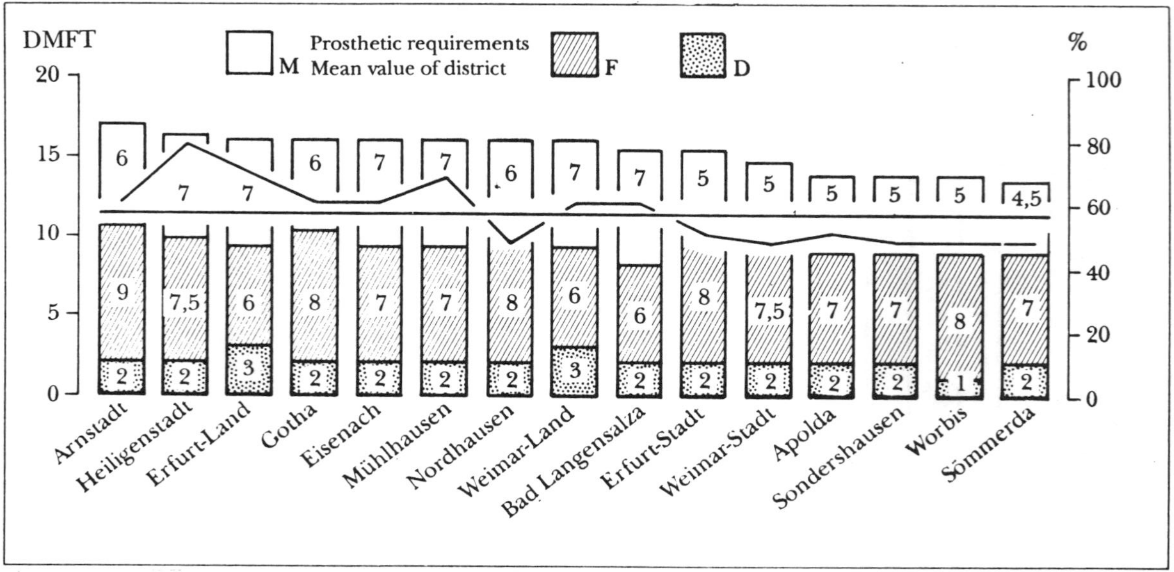

Fig. 1-7 Caries prevalence and mean number of filled and missing teeth (age group 35 to 44) in 15 districts of Erfurt county (— prosthetic requirements in districts and in the county —); requirement for removable (37%) and fixed prosthesis (21%).

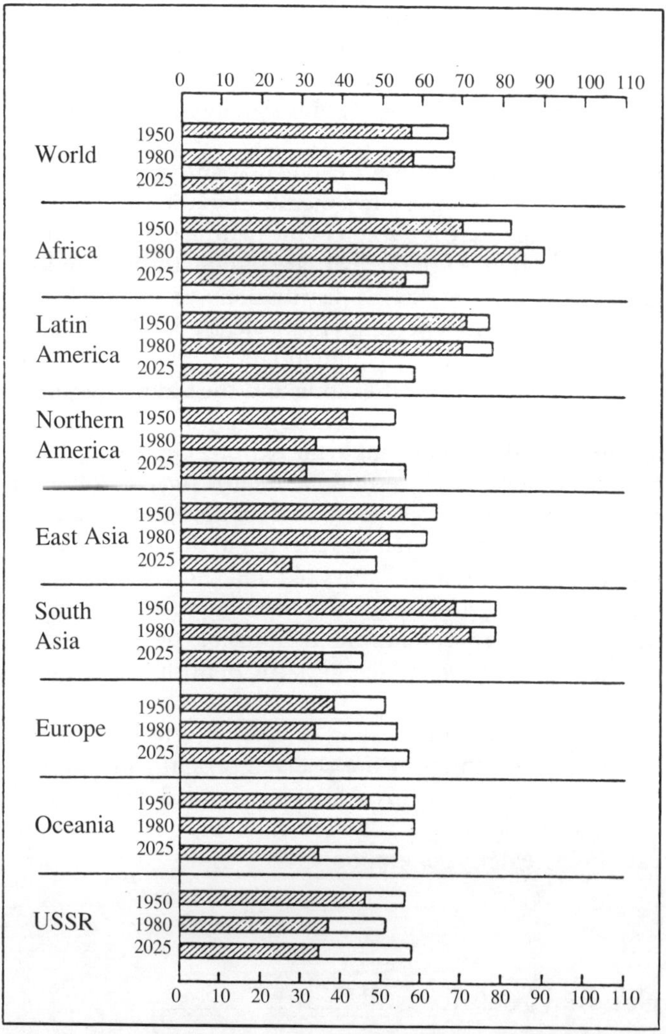

Fig. 1-8 Age dependency ratio for total, under 15 years, and over 65 years and over by region, medium variant, 1950, 1980 and 2025; shaded and white areas of bars represent the dependency ratios for under 15 years and over 65 years and over, respectively (United Nations, 1982).

sures, rahter than the progressive forms that require immediate therapeutic intervention by the dentist. The proportion of the population at greater risk of periodontitis is in the range 10% to 15% [36, 53], thus signalling a limited need for treatment.

Over the long term, therefore, one may anticipate a gradual displacement of conservative measures to the adult population and to life-long retention of the natural teeth. Given the present standard of the dental care system, the epidemiological change in oral disease distribution and in destruction of the dentition as it becomes more clearly visible in various nations, justifies the recommendation that a system of regular dental care for the aging and the elderly (geriatric [gerostomatological] dental care system) be initiated. Such a system could be analogous to the existing pediatric a dental care programme of prevention, treatment and follow-up care (school and adolescent dental care programmes). The need for this development is reflected in the comparison of populations less than 15 years old and those over 65 years (Fig 1-8), as they are expected to be in the year 2025, figures that, incidentally also indicate the possible prolongation of the time period over which geriatric dentistry services will be needed.

The major decision regarding such a projected profile line is determined in part by the availability of an efficient oral health care system and in part by an expanded, demographically and epidemiologically documented, need for dental care in the elderly generation.

National goals for oral health

Oral health care requires fundamental planning in conformity with the existing state of scientific knowledge and current national concepts for territorial levels. Such planning must lead to specific steps and prescribed stages (5 years) for targeted improvement of the oral health of defined groups of probands and must be examined for its actual effectiveness [33]. For example, the relatively good oral health of the population of the GDR, together with the level of oral health care available, provides a solid base for the qualitative further development of the dental care system. In fact, a future-oriented concept has been developed in co-operation with the Ministry of Health [6]. National goals for oral health, arising from and supported by epidemiological data, are goal oriented; these surpass the global indicators promulgated by the WHO and the FDI [16]. This is particularly true of the goals set for the year 2000, in terms of the number of natural teeth to be retained in the various age groups and in reduction of edentulousness:

	FDI's Global Goals	*GDR's National Goals*
Goal 1	50% of 5- and 6-year-olds to be caries free	60% of 5- and 6-year-olds to be caries free
Goal 2	Not more than 3 DMF teeth in 12-year-olds	Not more than 3 DMF teeth in 12-year-olds
Goal 3	Dentition retained by 80% of 18-year-olds	Dentition retained by 90% of 18-year-olds
Goal 4	Decrease edentulousness by 25% in the age group 35 to 44 years	24 functional natural teeth in the age group 35 to 44 years
Goal 5	25% reduction of edentulousness in the over-64 years age group	20 natural teeth in 50% of those over age 64, and not more than 25% edentulous

The formulation of such goals for oral health naturally raises the question of their attainability. The answer is particularly complicated for the senior citizen (over age 60) group. The

increase in natural teeth that may be ascribed to generational change is slow, expresses itself chiefly in the reduction of edentulousness, and diminishes after age 65 [5]. In setting strategic courses for care, one must start from national goals that arise from demographic reality and its development, from the epidemiologically determined demand for care, and the efficiency of the oral health care system. The attitude of the citizenry to oral health and its attitude to accepting dental care also must be considered.
The requirements for setting a new priority for geriatric dentistry may be formulated in this way:

- availability and continuous accessibility of an efficient oral health care delivery system, including an industrial dental care system;
- an adequate ratio of dental manpower to population (dentist: population ratio in the GDR in 1988 – 1:1280), in relation to the existing demand for care, and a sound ratio of dentists to dental auxiliaries (dental nurses in the GDR) and dental technicians;
- an enforced, complex preventive programme for children and adolescents [31], including organized early detection and treatment (including the treatment of dentofacial anomalies);
- availability of prosthetic care to the entire population;
- a fully developed prevention programme, including a recall system, comprehensive health education and prevention-oriented clinics, particularly for pregnant women and young mothers, health professionals, etc.

The 35- to 44-year-old age group is a special target because its members can be guided to the threshold of old age with better health conditions through specific measures taken over a period of 15 to 20 years. This requires that the existing "wait and see" attitude of dental care be converted to a "progressive" form [33], which should exist especially in the form of prevention-promoting contacts between the target group and the dental care collective.

Optimizing geriatric dental care

When considering the justified promotion of stepwise establishment of an organized geriatric dental care service, it must be recognized that the need is less a for a new professional and scientific approach than for a new level of health policy in terms of dental care for the elderly and the aged. In this sense, geriatric dentistry is another, specifically dental form to be integrated into existing official concepts for the social and medical care of the elderly population. From this point of view, specific and general requirements, with individual and collective aspects, may be set for geriatric dentistry. The chief problem here is found in the biologically determined diminution of the ability of the elderly individual to participate physically and psychologically in societal processes; this is disadvantageous to his health and to his well-being [23, 28]. That the infirmities and general symptoms of illness are more important to old and very old people than their reduced ability to speak and chew – which they may accept – is a fact that cannot be dismissed. Different care strategies are thus needed, as are the organizational requirements and possibilities that promote acceptance of dental care. For this reason, it is necessary to develop models for dental care in retirement homes and institutions that care for the aged (more than 172,000 beds in the GDR in 1987, according to the Statistisches Jahrbuch der DDR), and for the elderly who live in their own homes. These models must meet the limits imposed by the physically able and also those who are disabled to various degrees. Societal aspects also play a role. Finally, but not least important, resources such as the availability of academics, materials and time must be provided to provide the best outcome of care under the existing conditions.

Developmental strategies, based on epidemiological need, societal demand and individual acceptance, must be formulated for the dental care of the aged and their special requirements.

Bibliography

1. *Antalovská, Z.*
Symposium experimentální gerontologie. Česk Stomatol 86: 246, 1986.

2. *Armenio, G.*
Gerontologia stomatologica. Cortina, 1959.

3. *Arnljot, H.A. et al.*
Oral health care systems. An international collaborative study. World Health Organization, London: Quintessence Publishing Co., 1985.

4. *Balogh, K. et al.*
Gerostomatologie. Leipzig: Johann Ambrosius Barth Verlag, 1962.

5. *Bates, J.F. and Stafford G.D.*
Zahnärztliche Behandlung älterer Patienten. Berlin: Quintessenz-Verlag, 1986.

6. *Borutta, A. et al.*
Zahnärztliche Fortbildung. Eine Konzeption auf der Grundlage eines internationalen Effektivitätsvergleichs. Leipzig: Johann Ambrosius Barth Verlag, 1988 (Zahnärztliche Fortbildung. Neue Folge).

7. *Borutta, A., and Waurick, M.:*
Strategie der zahnärztlichen Betreuung in der DDR bis zum Jahr 2000 – Eine perspektivische Konzeption. Med Diss B, Erfurt, 1985.

8. *Bouma, J.*
On becoming edentulous. An investigation into the dental and behavioural reasons for full mouth extractions. Med Diss, Groningen, 1987.

9. *Branzi, A.*
Gerodontostomatologie. G. Geront. Suppl 9: 65, 1956.

10. *Breustedt, A.*
Aufgaben und Probleme der Gerostomatologie. Stomatol DDR 26: 517-525, 1976.

11. *Breustedt, A.*
Stomatologische Betreuung im höheren Lebensalter. Leipzig: Johann Ambrosius Barth Verlag, 1978.

12. *Bürger, M.*
Altern und Krankheit. 3. Aufl. Leipzig: Thieme, 1957.

13. *Butler, R.N.*
Therapeutic implications. In: Butler, R.N., and Bearn, A.G. (Eds.) The aging process. New York: Raven Press, 1984.

14. *Cecava, J.A. et al.*
Vývoj problematiky orofacialní gerontochirurgie v létech 1946-1980. Česk Stomatol 84: 252-258, 1984.

15. *Eitner, S.*
Praktische Gerohygiene. Handbuch der komplexen Betreuung im Alter. Dresden: Steinkopff, 1975.

16. *Fédération Dentaire Internationale.*
Global goals for oral health in the year 2000. Int Dent J 32: 74-77, 1982.

17. *Font, J.*
Gerostomatologia. Med Espan 32: 45, 1954.

18. *Frolkis, W.W.*
Mechanismen des Alterns. Berlin: Akademie-Verlag, 1975.

19. *Franks, A.S.T., and Hedegaord, B.:*
Geriatric Dentistry. Oxford: Blackwell Scientific Publications, 1973.

20. *Glass, R.L.*
The First International Conference on the Declining Prevalence of Dental Caries. J Dent Res 61: 1301-1383, 1982.

21. *Gorman, J.T.*
Recent advances in geriodontology. Dent Students Mag 21: Mo. 9, 1952.

22. *Höcker, M.*
Vergleichende stomatologische Erhebungen zur oralen Gesundheit in den verschiedenen Lebensaltern. Med Diss B, Berlin, 1983.

23. *Höcker, M.*
Stand und Perspektiven der Erhaltung der oralen Leistungsfähigkeit bis in das höhere und hohe Lebensalter. Wiss Z Humboldt-Univ. Berlin, Math-Nat-Wiss Reihe 34: 738-740, 1985.

24. *Holm-Pedersen, P. and Loe, H.*
Geriatric Dentistry. Copenhagen: Munksgaard, 1986.

25. *Imfeld, T.*
Alterszahnmedizin – Herausforderung der Zukunft. Swiss Dent 6: 7-8, 21-33, 1985.

26. *Jarcho, S.*
Blankaarts Dictionary, an index to 17th century medicine. Bull NYAcad Med 6: 568-577, 1982.

27. *Kail, B.I.P.*
Care for older people. Br Dent J 158: 320, 1985.

28. *Kandelmann, D., and Lepage, Y.*
Demographic, social and cultural factors influencing the elderly to seek dental treatment. Int Dent J 32: 360-370, 1982.

29. *Knak, G.*
Prothetisch-stomatologischer Versorgungsgrad und Versorgungsbedarf der Bevölkerung der Hauptstadt Berlins. Ergebnisse und Schlußfolgerungen einer repräsentativen Morbiditätsuntersuchung im Jahre 1972. Diss B, Berlin, 1974.

30. *Körber, E.*
Die zahnärztlich-prothetische Versorgung des älteren Menschen. München: Hanser, 1978.

31. *Künzel, W.*
Effects of comprehensive preventive programmes on oral health in children and juveniles in congested industrial areas. Int Dent J 34: 161-165, 1984.

32. *Künzel, W.*
The impact of changing patterns in dental diseases on practice of orthodontics. Int Dent J 37: 77-85, 1987.

33. *Künzel, W. et al.*
Empfehlungen zur perspektivischen Konzipierung der zahnärztlichen Betreuungsstrategie. Stomatol DDR 35: 101-112, 1985.

34. *Landt, H.*
Gerontologie. ZWR 94: 801-808, 1985.

35. *Leader*
Our elderly; top Priority. Br Dent J 157: 197, 1984.

36. *Löe, H.*
Principles of aetiology and pathogenesis governing the treatment of periodontal disease Int Dent J 33: 119-126, 1983.

37. *Massler, M.*
Geriatric dentistry: The problem. J Prosthet Dent 40: 324-325, 1978.

38. *Nascher, I.L.*
Geriatrics. New York Med J 90: 358, 1909.

39. *Peisachowitsch, I.M. et al.*
Gerontostomatologija. Kiew: Sdorowja, 1973.

40. *Renson, C.E. et al.*
Changing patterns of oral health and implications for oral health manpower: Part I. Int Dent J 35: 235-251, 1985.

41. *Ries, W.*
Zu den Beziehungen zwischen Altern und Krankheit. Z gesamte inn Med 31: 85-89, 1976.

42. *Rybnikow, N.A.*
Das Problem der Psychologie des Alterns (Russ.) Zurnal Psikhologii i Psikotekniki 2: 16-32, 1919/29.

43. *Sauerwein, E. (Hrsg.)*
Gerontostomatologie. Stuttgart, New York: Thieme, 1981.

44. *Thomae, H., and Lehr, U.*
Eine Botschaft der Internationalen Association für Gerontologie an die UN-Weltkonferenz über Probleme des Altern. Z Gerontol 15: 132-137, 1982.

45. *Thomas, B.O.A.*
"Gerodontology": the study of changes in oral tissues associated with aging. J Am Dent Assoc 33: 207, 1946.

46. *Tschebotarew, D.F. and N.V. Verzhikovskaya:*
Problems of health and position of the elderly in socialist countries of eastern Europe. Z Alternsforsch 36: 437-472, 1981.

47. *United Nations*
Demographic indicators of countries: estimates and projections as assessed in 1980. New York, 1982.

48. *United Nations*
World population prospects. Estimates and projections as assessed in 1984. Population studies No. 98, New York, 1986.

49. *Walther, R.G.*
Stomatologische Morbiditätsuntersuchung nach über zwanzigjähriger Fluoridierung des Trinkwassers von Karl-Marx-Stadt bei den Erwachsenen der Bevölkerung – Ermittlung des Betreuungsbedarfs und Konzeption eines Betreuungsprogramms. Diss B, Erfurt 1986.

50. *Waurick, M.*
Epidemiologie marginaler Erkrankungen – Grundlage einer präventiv orientierten Betreuungsstrategie. Zahn- Mund- Kieferheilkd 74: 555-562, 1986.

51. *Wilke, G.*
Studien über die Beziehungen zwischen Alter und stomatologischen Befunden im biologisch-soziologisch-psychohygienischen Aspekt. Med Diss, Berlin, 1969.

52. *WHO*
Protecting the health of the elderly. Public Health in Europe 18. Copenhagen: WHO Regional Office for Europe, 1983.

53. *Waurick, M.*
Oraler Gesundheitszustand ausgewählter Probandengruppen. Stomatol DDR 35: 71-81, 1985.

54. *Zakson, M.L.*
Prothetische Gerontostomatologie (Ortopediceskaja gerontostomatologija) Kiev, 1986.

55. *Ziegler, J.E.*
Geriodontics. J South California Dent Assoc 24: 29, 1956.

Part II Clinical Aspects

Chapter 2
Does Life-long Retention of Natural Teeth Imply Higher Risks of Caries and Periodontitis?

Annerose Borutta, Roswitha Heinrich and Walter Künzel

As a result of progress in medicine, the average life expectancy has increased significantly in industrialized nations. This has led to a larger percentage of elderly and old persons; beyond the turn of the century, estimates indicate that persons over age 65 years will make up 20% of the population[3]. Oral health care systems must adjust to this altered demographic situation; adequate care systems appropriate to the population must be developed. A prerequisite to this process, given the numerous social and geriatric problems, however, are data describing the distribution and severity of oral diseases. Because of the difficulties associated with recording of data in this population, only a few representative studies of the prevalence of caries and periodontal disease exist. Information about the oral condition of the elderly population is important, however, for planning of appropriate care programmes; at present, only the average adult population data can be used. Extension of comprehensive preventive programmes to entire populations makes reduction in the high rate of edentulousness in the middle-aged, and life-long retention of increasing

numbers of natural teeth possible. Age-related involution and inflammation changes of the marginal periodontium, which elicit the increased risk of root caries associated with exposure of the cementum, cannot be excluded.
Taking the anticipated demographic and epidemiological developments into consideration, two tentative conclusions may be advanced:

1. The retention of natural teeth to advanced age is accompanied by increased prevalence of diseases of the marginal periodontium and dental hard tissue, particularly of the root surfaces.
2. Integration of prevention-oriented care programmes appropriate to the age group in all dental specialties makes the risk of morbidity of the dominating oral diseases controllable.

The prevention-directed oral health care strategy developed for the GDR is oriented to 20 functional teeth in 50% of all persons over age 65 years in the year 2000. In addition, the proportion of edentulous persons should not exceed 25%[6].
The results of the ICS-I* and subsequent national studies show that the oral health status of the adult population offers a favourable basis for attainment of these targets. The population is characterized by having a large number of natural teeth, average caries prevalence and almost complete freedom from edentulousness.
As to the marginal periodontium, studies made in representative samples of 35- to 44-year-old probands made with the aid of the CPITN show that reversible inflammation states predominate in this age group. Calculus and shallow pockets were the most frequent attributes (Table 2-1). Extrapolating these findings to the number of segments (Table 2-2) shows that five pathological characteristics exist, on average. A total of 0.6 segments could not be evaluated, owing to premature extraction of the index or comparison

* International Collaborative Study of Dental Manpower Systems

Table 2-1 Periodontal health status; percentage distribution of probands (Age 35 to 44 years)

Location	N	H Healthy periodontium	B Bleeding	C Calculus	P1 4 to 5 mm pocket	P2 ≥ 6 mm pocket
Berlin	100	0	16.49	39.56	37.36	6.60
Cottbus	100	0	6.06	32.32	54.55	7.07
Dresden	100	0	3.00	30.00	62.00	5.00
Erfurt	100	0	18.81	53.47	23.76	3.96
Frankfurt /Oder	100	0	1.01	25.25	39.40	15.15
Gera	71	0	8.57	58.57	28.57	4.29
Halle	79	0	2.56	37.18	51.28	8.98
K-Marx-Stadt	47	0	12.77	42.55	36.17	8.51
Leipzig	88	0	14.12	48.24	31.76	5.88
Magdeburg	100	0	2.04	37.78	42.85	17.34
Neubrandenburg	100	0	11.22	34.70	50.00	4.08
Potsdam	96	0	8.38	53.13	35.42	2.08
Rostock	100	0	12.00	48.00	38.00	2.00
Suhl	80	0	6.41	53.85	33.34	6.41

teeth, and only 0.4 were free of inflammation. In the five segments of dentition having characteristics of pathology, bleeding and calculus dominated. Shallow pocket depths were demonstrated in only one segment, on average. Pathological pocket depths, those deeper than 5.5 mm, were less frequent. These studies indicate that oral hygiene instruction must be emphasized, followed by scaling of an average of three segments. In contrast, comprehensive care appears indicated in only 7%± 2 to 17% of probands, based on the rarity of deep pockets (Table 2-3).

The limited data related to probands over age 65 years available at present show that the percentage of advanced periodontal disease increases when compared to middle-aged persons, but is still below 25% (Fig. 2-1). This provides supplemental information for the GDR about periodontal health status in the year 2000. Accordingly, not more than 10% of

Table 2-2 Average number of segments per person

Study area	N	0 Healthy Periodon-tium	1+2+3+4 higher or bleeding score	2+3+4 higher or calculus score	3+4 higher shallow pock-et or score	4 deep pocket	x fewer than 2 teeth
Berlin	100	0.22	4.55	2.51	1.11	0.07	1.23
Cottbus	100	0.12	5.53	3.78	1.45	0.08	0.24
Dresden	100	0.26	4.91	3.49	1.52	0.05	0.83
Erfurt	100	0.48	5.09	2.26	0.42	0.06	0.44
Frankfurt/O	100	0.16	5.32	4.09	1.93	0.17	0.52
Gera	71	0.50	5.07	3.13	0.57	0.05	0.69
Halle	79	0.12	5.38	3.31	1.25	0.13	0.50
Karl-Marx-Stadt	47	0.26	5.40	3.28	0.45	0.13	0.36
Leipzig	88	0.41	5.26	2.61	0.90	0.12	0.31
Magdeburg	100	0.12	5.03	3.67	1.71	0.20	0.64
Neubrandenburg	100	0.23	5.15	2.97	1.28	0.04	0.61
Potsdam	96	0.26	4.45	2.53	0.68	0.02	1.31
Rostock	100	0.29	5.15	2.72	0.77	0.02	0.56
Suhl	80	0.07	4.71	2.63	0.72	0.09	1.23

Table 2-3 Periodontal health status of persons aged 35 to 44 years in various regions of the GDR

Location	N	Oral Hygiene instruction % TN 1	Scaling % TN 2	Complex treatment % TN 3
Berlin	100	100.00	97.97	17.34
Cottbus	100	40.00	93.94	7.07
Dresden	100	100.00	97.00	5.00
Erfurt	100	100.00	81.18	3.96
Frankfurt/O	100	80.81	79.80	15.15
Gera	71	100.00	91.43	4.29
Halle	79	100.00	97.44	8.96
Karl-Marx-Stadt	47	100.00	87.23	8.51
Leipzig	88	100.00	85.88	5.83
Magdeburg	100	100.00	97.97	17.34
Neubrandenburg	100	100.00	88.78	4.08
Potsdam	96	100.00	90.63	2.08
Rostock	100	100.00	88.00	2.00
Suhl	80	100.00	93.59	6.41

Table 2-4 Prevalence of root caries in the population of Erfurt (N = 963)

Age (years)	Women (%)	Men (%)
25 to 34	17.9	11.7
35 to 44	33.7	63.0
45 to 54	59.6	56.6
55 to 64	59.0	47.5
Total	40.2	42.7

the over age 65 population should have one or more segments of dentition requiring comprehensive periodontal treatment[2,6].

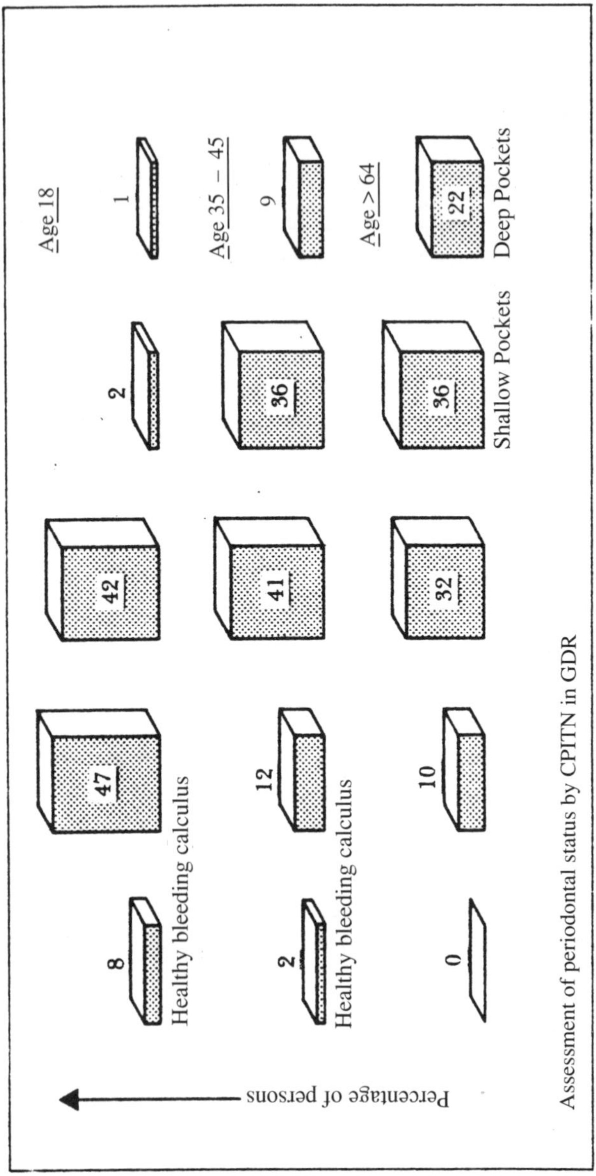

Fig. 2-1 Periodontal health status in different age groups of the GDR population by CPITN.

Only limited information about the frequency and prevalence of root caries, including risk of disease and the intraoral preference pattern, is available internationally. Prevalence data vary between 15% and 83%, arising from different study populations and different methods of evaluation; such differences make comparisons between studies impossible.[1,5,8-10] Initial studies have been carried out in the GDR on the amount of care required for treatment of root caries. These show that on average, 40% of adults have a carious or restored root surface. Frequency increases with increasing age, parallel with periodontal disease, and reaches 60% in 64-year-olds (Table 2-4). The exposed root surface appears at first glance to determine the risk, but in fact, the age-related increase in recession, with an analogous increase in caries, is decisive. The hypothetically assumed age dependence of risk underlying the root caries index (RCI) of *Katz*[4] must be rejected. While the number of surfaces with gingival recession, caries or restorations or both, and carious or restored root surfaces increases by more than a factor of 10, the risk of occurrence, measured by the RCI, remains nearly constant (Tables 2-5 and 2-6). This inclusive age independence results from the synchronous increase of at risk – diseased and restored root surfaces, with preferential attack of the mandibular molars and maxillary canines.

Analysis of the present epidemiological situation leads inevitably to the conclusion that neither prevalence nor severity of periodontal disease or root caries rate in the elderly provide insurmountable problems in care. The brisk loss of an average of ten teeth, from the 35- to 44-year cohort to that aged 55 to 64 years, and the relatively high rate of edentulousness of those over age 65 is in stark contrast to the present pattern of oral disease prevalence. Thus, inadequate oral health care must be recognized as the immediate cause of the unsatisfactory oral health of elderly citizens.

In principle, however, the established dental care system of the GDR appears to satisfy the demand for functional retention of the dentition into advanced old age. It cannot be imagined that the dentition must be completely free of patho-

Table 2-5 Prevalence of root caries by number and affected teeth in relation to age and sex

Age (years)		No. of teeth		No. of teeth with root caries		Average of teeth with root caries	
		Female	Male	Female	Male	Female	Male
25 to 34	$\bar{x}$	25.8	26.9	0.4	0.4	1.6	2.2
	s	± 4.5	± 3.4	± 1.1	± 1.7	± 4.6	± 9.7
35 to 44	$\bar{x}$	23.2	23.8	1.0	2.6	5.0	11.6
	s	± 6.2	± 5.3	± 1.9	± 4.0	± 11.3	± 17.3
45 to 54	$\bar{x}$	20.1	20.0	1.7	2.5	10.6	15.0
	s	± 9.0	± 7.4	± 2.1	± 3.1	± 14.7	± 19.6
55 to 64	$\bar{x}$	13.0	13.2	1.7	1.3	17.6	11.3
	s	± 8.5	± 9.2	± 2.1	± 1.8	± 26.3	± 16.8

Table 2-6 Number of root surfaces with gingival recessions, caries and/or fillings (percentage of all existing surfaces) and RCI depending on age and sex

Age (years)	Root surfaces with gingival recession, caries and/or restorations		Root surfaces with caries and/or restorations		RCI	
	Women	Men	Women	Men	Women	Men
25 to 34	3.85	6.0	0.44	0.6	11.44	9.4
35 to 44	11.9	25.8	1.2	3.2	10.5	12.4
45 to 54	27.7	37.4	2.9	5.0	10.5	13.3
55 to 64	42.3	58.1	5.5	3.5	12.9	5.9

logical changes. That goal would be unrealistic, because the natural aging process is accompanied by structural changes. Instead, the demands made of oral health care providers will change qualitatively. For that reason, geriatric dentistry cannot be limited to prosthetic dentistry alone. Care of the elderly requires appropriate use of all dental specialty disciplines.

Bibliography

1. *Banting, D.W., Ellen, R.P. and Fillery, E.D.*
Prevalence of root surface caries among institutionalized older persons
Community Dent Oral Epidemiol 8: 84-88, 1980

2. *Gängler, P. et al.*
Assessment of periodontal disease and dental caries in a population survey using the CPITN, GPM/T and DMF/T indices.
Community Dent Oral Epidemiol 16: 236-239, 1988.

3. *Imfeld, T.*
Altersmedizin – Herausforderung der Zukunft. Swiss Dent. 6: 21-33, 1985.

4. *Katz, R.V.*
A method for scoring and reporting root caries in epidemiologic studies.
J Dent Res 58: 389, 1979.

5. *Katz, R.V., Newitter, D.A. and Clive, J.M.*
Root caries prevalence in adult dental patients.
J Dent Res 64: 293, 1985.

6. *Künzel, W. et al.*
Empfehlungen zur perspektivischen Konzipierung der zahnärztlichen Betreuungsstrategie.
Stomatol DDR 35: 101-112, 1985.

7. *Künzel, W., Borutta, A. and Waurick, M.*
Bestimmung und Veränderung des periodontalen Behandlungsbedarfs in der Population.
Forschungsbericht HFR Karies und Periodontalerkrankungen M 27 Erfurt, 1988.

8. *Lohse, W.G., Carter, H.G. and Brunelle, I.A.*
The prevalence of root surface caries in a military population.
Milit Med 142: 700-703, 1977.

9. *Ravald, N. and Hamp, E.E.*
Prediction of root surface caries in patients treated for advanced periodontal disease.
J Clin Period 8: 400-414, 1980.

10. *Schamschula, R.G. et al.*
Prevalence and interrelationships of root caries in Lufa, Papua-New Guinea.
Community Dent Oral Epidemiol 12: 295-304, 1974.

11. *Vehkalahti, M. et al.*
Prevalence of root caries in adult Finnish population.
Community Dent Oral Epidemiol 11: 188-190, 1983.

Chapter 3
Clinical Aspects of Root Surface Caries

Vito Vrbic

Compared with coronal caries, root surface caries (RSC) has received much less attention and many of its aspects are still unclear. This is the usual consensus of any major meeting devoted to this topic, from the first root caries symposium in Boston in 1985 to the root caries symposium organized concurrently with the 34th ORCA Congress in Budapest in 1987. In the conclusions the participants generally underscore the need for further research into the aetiology, development and treatment of root caries.

Aetiology and prevention of root surface caries

Whereas the microbial picture of coronal caries is dominated by *Streptococcus mutans*, *Actinomyces* species are usually predominant in root caries lesions.

Jordan [13] points out that early investigations of root caries in experimental animals have provided valuable insight into some of the dieto-bacterial interactions involved. However, these findings have not been completely validated at the human level. It seems that interactions between oral bacteria and other factors involved in the development of root surface caries may be broader in scope and more difficult to interpret than the bacterial activities which result in coronal caries. Additional clinical studies are needed to compare the microbial populations and their activities on intact and caries cemental surfaces.

To prevent a disease, it is necessary to understand its aetiology. No root caries can take place unless there has been loss of periodontal attachment with or without gingival recession. Prevention of root caries therefore involves prevention of periodontal disease (by personal oral hygiene and use of antimicrobial agents), avoidance of sucrose, drinking of optimally fluoridated water and the appropriate use of topical fluoride agents. The concentration of fluoride in the outer layer of the root surface increases with increasing levels of fluoride in the water supply as well as with advancing age [5]. Epidemiological data indicate that lifelong residence in a fluoridated community is associated with a highly significant reduction in the prevalence of root caries or root fillings at all ages [27].

Besides oral hygiene instruction and dietary advice, topical fluoride application is one of the most effective root caries preventive treatments. The fluoride agents that have been used with success include: 1.1% sodium fluoride gel, 0.4% stannous fluoride gel and 0.05% sodium fluoride rinse [19].

Demineralization and remineralization of root surface caries

Relatively few studies have investigated natural demineralization and remineralization of the RSC lesion, compared to lesions in enamel. Dentine and cementum are less mineralized than enamel and dissolve more rapidly in acid [6]. Artificial lesions in roots were found to be deeper than lesions in enamel when formed in the same teeth under the same conditions [22].

When sound cementum is exposed to the oral environment it rapidly acquires an organic pellicle and then frequently takes up minerals from the saliva to form a thin hypermineralized surface layer of about 50 µm [26]. Hypermineralization of dentine has also been observed deep within a root surface lesion [29].

Fluoride appears at significant levels in cementum and increases both with age and in the presence of fluoridated water [2]. Fluoride contributes to the formation of the hypermineralized layer on the root surface [7]. Some hypermineralization of the surface might also result from the acquisition of trace elements, such as zinc, silver and tin [9]. Although active research into the remineralization of RSC is still in the initial stage, it is evident that lesions on the root can be partially remineralized and that lesions on the root can be partially remineralized and that fluoride will enhance the process [18].

Prevalence and definitions of root surface caries

Accurate data on the prevalence of root caries are lacking. Data are available only for a small number of countries (USA, Finland, Sweden, India, New Guinea, Egypt). They are often not comparable, since the studies were performed in different age groups and different methodologies were employed for the diagnosis of root caries lesions. In the studies reviewed by *Vehkalahti* [28] the prevalence rates generally ranged from 20% to 40%, depending on the age of the study population and the definition of root caries used by the author. Three different definitions where used: primary caries on the root surface; primary and secondary caries on the root surfaces; all filled and carious root surfaces. The frequency of root caries has been shown to be proportional to age. A greater prevalence for men than for women has been reported in several studies[28]. Data on the location and distribution of root caries in the oral cavity reported by different authors show considerable discrepancies. *Katz* et al. [14] found the greatest number of lesions on mandibular molars, followed by mandibular premolars and maxillary canines. *Hix* and *O'Leary* [11] observed root caries to be most common in mandibular molars and premolars. *Banting* et al. [1] demonstrated that the majority of root caries lesions were situated on proximal surfaces and that most teeth were affected on one surface only. *Katz* et al. [14] reported that buccal surfaces in the mandible and interproximal surfaces in the maxilla exhibited the highest frequencies of root caries.

Various definitions have been proposed to describe carious lesions located on the root. *Hix* and *O'Leary* [11], for example, defined root caries as "a cavitation or softened area in the root surface, generally well established, discoloured and characterized by penetration and destruction of underlying dentine". *Hazen* et al. [10] defined root caries as "soft, progressive, destructive lesions either totally confined to the root surface or involving the undermining of enamel at the cemento-enamel junction, but with firm clinical evidence that the lesion initiated on the root surface". *Katz* [16] has proposed six conventions to ensure more accurate and consistent diagnosis of root caries in clinical research.

The difference in tactile sensation between sound and carious enamel is far greater than that for cementum or dentine. Therefore, a special explorer or probe is required to detect root caries lesions. An explorer of this type was developed by *Newitter* and *Katz* [20]. Root caries is diagnosed if the point of the explorer is inserted easily into the carious area with moderate finger pressure[11] or when the explorer easily enters the lesion and displays some resistance to withdrawal (*Banting* et al., 1985).

Severity of surface caries and appropriate treatment

It is important that not all root surfaces are covered entirely with cementum. In as many as 30% of teeth, the cementum and enamel do not meet [23], and therefore caries at the cemento-enamel junction may start directly in the dentine. As the cariogenic attack progresses into the dentine, the more highly mineralized peritubular dentine is demineralized more rapidly than intertubular dentine [25].

When the root surface is covered with cementum, it is generally accepted that the initial destruction that occurs upon a cariogenic challenge to the cementum is a loss of mineral [9]. However, an *in vitro* experiment has shown that the proteolytic enzyme papain can result in matrix destruction, with total tissue loss from the human root [15].

Root surface lesions are classified according to shape, extent and depth. The most sensible classification appears to be that of *Billings* et al. (1982), which distinguishes between incipient, shallow, cavitated and pulpal lesions (root caries severity index), also taking into account various treatment categories. Cavity preparation on the root differs from that on the crown, mainly with respect to cavity depth and design. Often an extensively modified preparation is required, especially when root caries extends occluso-gingivally or circumferentially around the tooth. Because of these peculiarities, amalgam is not always a suitable filling material. In addition, composite resins should not be used since etching is inappropriate and does not produce microretention. More suitable for use are dentine adhesives with composite resin, although the long-term clinical efficiency of these materials has not been established.

Glass ionomer cements have been used successfully for the treatment of root surface erosions. This material adheres to enamel and dentine by means of physicochemical bonding [12]. Its retention on the root surface seems to be very good (*Billings* et al, 1985).

Further improvements are expected from a new method of bonding resin-based filling materials to glass ionomer cements by prior acid etching of the cement surface. Some authors term such cement »replacement dentine« [17]. *In vivo* evaluation of glass ionomer cements has demonstrated absence of irreversible pulpal response [21]. *Garcia* et al. [8] report that these materials have no adverse effect on gingival tissues. Another advantage of glass ionomer cement is that it contains fluoride, which is taken up and retained for extended periods in enamel and dentine [24]. Since fluoride is released into the surroundings, no evidence of recurrent caries has been found around the margins of glass ionomer restored root caries lesions (*Billings* et al., 1985). Because of these attributes, glass ionomer cement should be considered the material of choice for restoring root surface dental caries.
Guidelines for the treatment or restoration of root surface dental caries, according to *Billings* [4], are given below:

Grade I (incipient) lesions – smoothing with polishing discs and topically applied fluoride.
Grade II (shallow) lesions – recontouring and smoothing with abrasives, prophylaxis pastes, polishing discs, fine diamonds and topically applied fluoride.
Grade III (cavitated) lesions – restoration with glass ionomer cement and topically applied fluoride.

The present epidemiological data indicate that root caries increases with age. Since the number of people in older population categories is increasing, root caries may be expected to become more and more common. This prediction is also supported by the anticipated increase in tooth longevity due to the declining caries prevalence in children and adolescents. Thus root caries is likely to become a major health problem in dentistry. Our present knowledge of root caries is insufficient and more research is needed into every aspect of the disease. It is especially important that we obtain more information about the prevalence of the disease, so that we can follow its trend.

Bibliography

1. *Banting, D.W., Ellen, R.P. and Fillery, E.D.*
Prevalence of root surface caries among institutionalized older persons. Community Dent Oral Epidemiol 8: 84-88, 1980.

2. *Banting, D.W. and Stamm, J.W.*
Effects of age and length of exposure to fluoridated water on root surface fluoride concentration. Clinical Preventive Dentistry 4(4): 3-7, 1982.

3. *Banting, D.W.*
Epidemiology of root caries. Gerontology 5: 5-11, 1986.

4. *Billings, J.*
Restoration of carious lesions of the root. Gerontology 5: 43-49, 1986.

5. *Brudevold, F., Steadman, L.T. and Smith, F.A.*
Inorganic and organic components of tooth structure. Ann NY Acad Sci 85: 119-132, 1960.

6. *Feagin, F.F.*
Mineral flux of surface enamel and root surfaces in acidified gelatin gels. J Oral Pathol 13: 497-504, 1984.

7. *Furseth, R.*
A study of experimentally exposed and fluoride treated dental cementum in pigs. Acta Odontol Scand 28: 833-850, 1970.

8. *Garcia, R., Cafesse, R.G. and Charbeneau, G.T.*
Gingival tissue response to restoration of deficient cervical contours using a glass-ionomer material. A 12-month report. Prosthet Dent 46: 393-398, 1981.

9. *Hals, E. and Selvig, K.A.*
Correlated electron probe microanalysis and microradiography of carious and normal dental cementum. Caries Res 11: 62-75, 1977.

10. *Hazen, S.P., Chilton, N.W. and Mumma Jr, R. D.*
The problem of root caries 3. A clinical study. J Dent Res 1972; 50: 219

11. *Hix, J.O. and O'Leary, T.J.*
The relationship between cemental caries oral hygiene status and fermentable carbohydrate intake. J. Periodontol 47: 398-404, 1976.

12. *Hotz, P. et al.*
The bonding of glass ionomer cements to metal and tooth substrates, Br Dent J 142: 41-47, 1977.

13. *Jordan, V.*
Microbial etiology of root surface caries. Gerontology 5: 13-20, 1986.

14. *Katz, R.V. et al.*
Prevalence and intraoral distribution of root caries in an adult population. Caries Res 16: 265-271, 1982.

15. *Katz, S. and Park, K.K.*
Factors involved in root caries formation J Dent Res 63: 222, 1983.

16. *Katz, R.*
The clinical identification of root caries. Gerontology 5: 21-24, 1986.

17. *McLean, J.W. Prosser, H.J. and Wilson, A.D.*
The use of glass-ionomer cements in bonding composite resins to dentine. Br Dent 15: 410-414, 1985.

18. *Melberg, J.R.*
Demineralization and remineralization of root surface caries. Gerontology 5: 25-31, 1986.

19. *Newbrun, E.*
Prevention of root caries. Gerontology 5: 33-34, 1986.

20. *Newitter, D.A., Katz, R.V. and Clive, J.M.*
Detection of root caries: Sensitivity and specificity of a modified explorer. Gerondontist 1: 65-67, 1985.

21. *Pameijer, C.H., Segal, E. and Richardson, J.*
Pulpal response to a glass ionomer cement in primates. Prosthet Dent 46: 36-40, 1981.

22. *Phankosol, P. et al.*
Depth of penetration of *in vitro* root surface lesions. J Dent Res 64: 987-899, 1985.

23. *Ramsey, D.J. and Ripa, L.W.*
Enamel prism orientation and enamel cementum relationship in the cervical region of premolar teeth. Br Dent J 126: 165-167, 1969.

24. *Retief, D.H. et al.*
Enamel and cementum fluoride uptake from a glass ionomer cement. Caries Res 18: 250-257, 1984.

25. *Selvig, K.A.*
Effect of fluoride on the acid solubility of human dentine. Arch Oral Biol 14: 1297-1310, 1968.

26. *Selvig, K.A. and Hals, E.*
Periodontally diseased cementum studied by correlated microradiography, electron probe analysis and electron microscopy. J Periodont Res 12: 419-429, 1977.

27. *Stamm, J.W. and Bantin, D.W.*
Comparison of root caries prevalence in adults with life-long residence in fluoridated and non-fluoridated communities. J Dent Res 59: 405, 1980.

28. *Vehkalahti, M.*
Occurrence of root caries and factors related to it. Academic dissertation, Helsinki, 1987.

29. *Westbrook, J.L. et al.*
Root surface caries: a clinical histopathologic and microradiographic investigation. Caries Res 8: 249-255, 1974.

Chapter 4
Epidemiological Evaluation of Edentulousness and the Need for Prosthodontic Care

E. Lenz

The increase in the proportion of aged and elderly in the population of European nations and experience with existing dental care programmes for the older population underline the need for systematic geriatric dental care oriented to the maintenance of the oral structures. Such a system remains to be devised, both in its organizational form and its specific direction.

The scientific basis for these requirements is the understanding of the oral diseases afflicting individuals aged 55 years or more, and the dental care level provided to this group. Frequency of tooth loss and the quantity and quality of prosthodontic care is of particularly great significance. Representative epidemiological studies of the oral health status in five European nations have been provided in the International Collaborative Study of Dental Manpower Systems (ICS) [12]. These studies include the adult population aged 35 to 44 years and, with DMF/T values of 14 to 26, indicate caries as the chief cause of damage to the dentition and tooth loss. The frequency of tooth loss varies greatly in this age group in various nations (average 5 to 14 missing teeth). It is lowest in Leipzig (GDR), with a rate of 4.7, thus indica-

Table 4-1 Epidemiological studies of edentulousness

Authors	(Year)	Age groups (yrs)	Group examined	Number
Taege and Fabrizius	(1967)	15 to 60	Factory employees	1234
Amreihn and Glöckner	(1968)	17 to 70	rural-population	3987
Götsch and Neubert	(1969)	17 to 70	Mass x-ray study (rural district)	1785
Dorsch and Laetzsch	(1973)	20 to 81	mass x-ray study	3576
Knak, et al.	(1975)	18 to 100	urban population	3853
Hoefig	(1974)	50 to 88	urban dental patients	8641
Kaden	(1980)	18 to 71	urban and rural dental patients	1599
Sandig	(1984)	20 to 75	urban dental patients	1042
Scholz	(1986)	24 to 75	rural dental patients	978

ting a functionally satisfactory dental status. Edentulousness (Leipzig: 0.5%) has no epidemiological role in this age group. The results of the ICS do not permit prediction of need for dental care in advanced age, however; instead, representatively comprehensive epidemiological investigations are needed in pre-retirement and retired age groups. Such studies remain to be done.

Review of the literature, however, provides some epidemiological data that include populations over age 60, collected over the past 20 years (Table 4-1 a, b). These studies involve widely differing samples, e.g. industrial plant workers, participants in serial radiographic studies and dental patients, all at geographically diverse locations; as a rule, such studies are not representative.

Epidemiology of tooth loss

Figure 4-1 a and b show the average numbers of missing teeth in relation to age of probands, as calculated from eight epidemiological studies. They indicate clearly the increase in tooth loss between age 40 and age 60. On average, 10 teeth are lost in this period, so that at age 60 years, 12 to 17 natural teeth remain. Sex differences in tooth loss, <2%, are very small [1, 8]. More recent studies [8, 16, 17] agree that a tendency exists toward retention of more natural teeth in those currently aged over 60 years. These results represent data collected in groups of dental patients; thus, they do not demonstrate a change in morbidity.

Evaluation of frequency of edentulousness is also possible in studies by *Götsch* et al. [7] and *Höefig* [8]. A summarization of their data (Fig. 4-2) shows a constant increase in edentulousness in the 6th and 7th decades of life, which appears initially – and at twice the frequency – in the maxilla. Men are edentulous in the maxilla at a rate 2% to 5% greater than women; the difference is very small in the mandible.

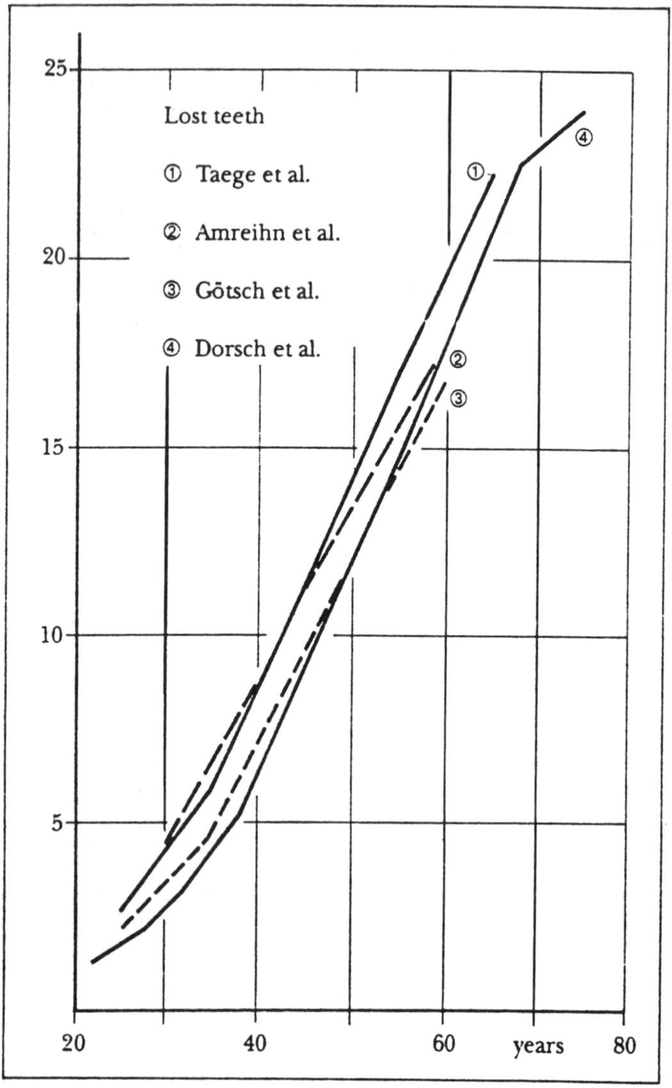

Fig. 4-1 a Mean number of natural teeth depending on age; date according to Table 4-1.

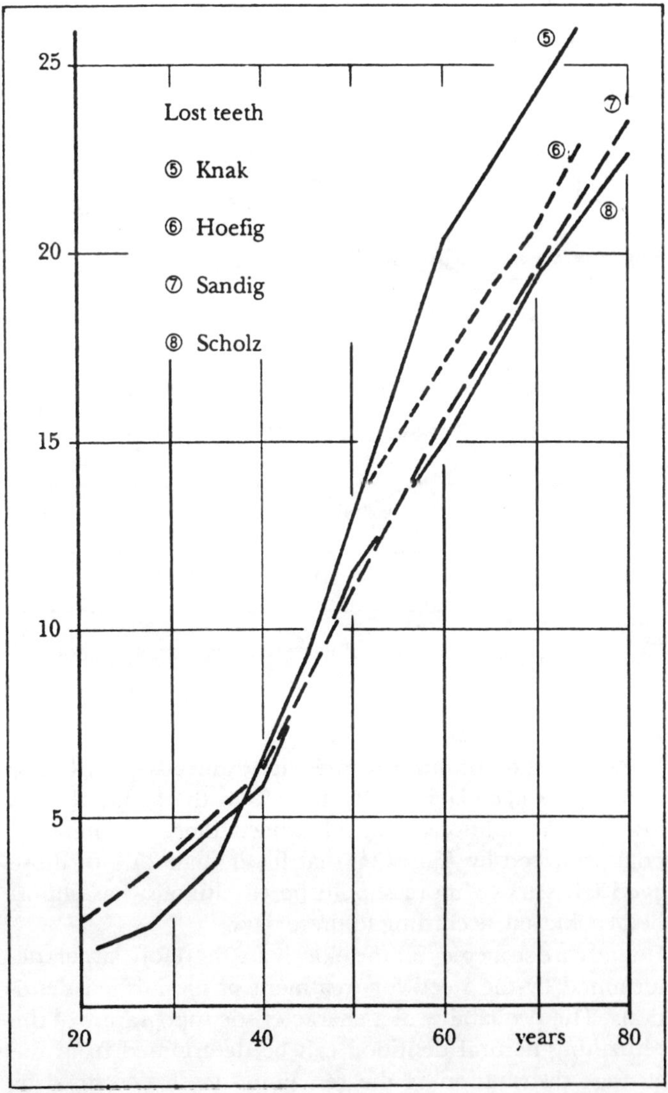

Fig. 4-1 b Mean number of natural teeth depending on age; date according to Table 4-1.

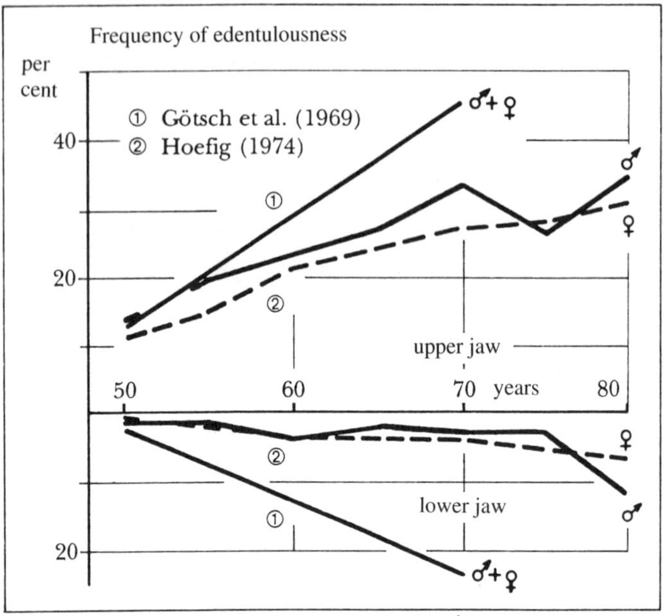

Fig. 4-2 Frequency of edentulousness in age groups about 50 years.

Maximum edentulousness rates at advanced age, 30% to 50% in the maxilla and 15% to 25% in the mandible, are lower than traditional clinical expectations. The national goal proposed by *Künzel* [11], that fewer than 25% of those aged 64 years or more should be edentulous, has almost been achieved, according to these data.

Dental care strategies for the elderly are therefore largely determined by the need for treatment of diminished dentitions. The probability of a characteristic topography of the remaining natural dentition can be determined from the average distribution of the remaining teeth described by *Hoefig* [8] (Fig 4-3). For the age groups 65 to 69 years and 75 to 79 years, parallel curves are found; both demonstrate do-

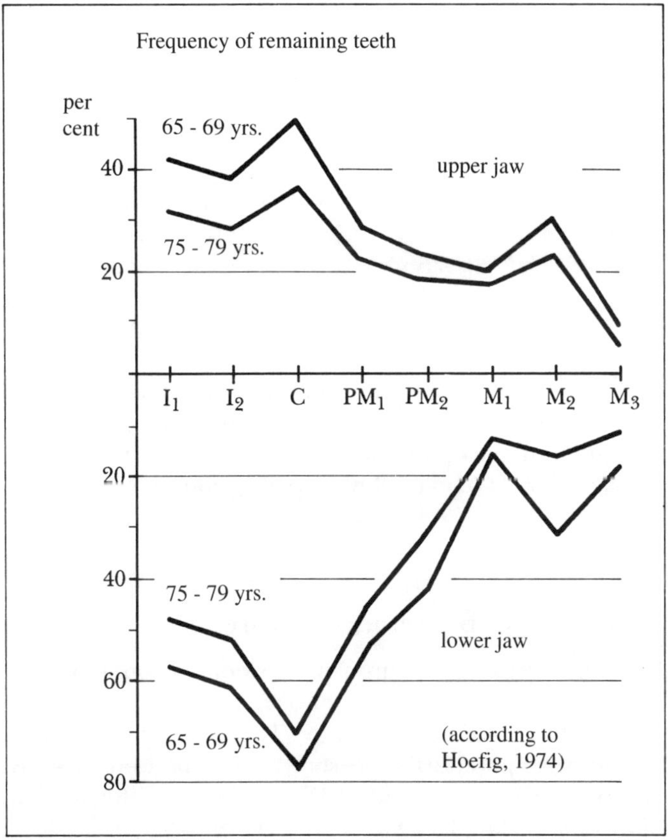

Fig. 4-3 Distribution of frequency of existing natural teeth in age groups 65-69 and 75-79[8].

minance of anterior teeth in the remaining dentition. This means that the following can be expected until the end of the 8th decade of life:

– anterior remaining teeth (including the first premolar) in the mandible in approximately 50% of patients;
– mandible canines in 70%;
– incisors and canines in more than 40% of the maxillas.

These estimates of the epidemiology of tooth loss lead to the following conclusions:

1. The frequency of edentulousness is relatively low in the geriatric population (<50% in the maxilla; <25% in the mandible).
2. Some remaining natural teeth can be anticipated well into old age (maxilla: >40%; mandible: >50%).
3. A preventive prosthodontic strategy is possible and necessary well into old age. Its emphasis should be on maintenance of the remaining teeth and functional support of the prosthesis.
4. The relatively large proportion of natural teeth present in the elderly demands epidemiological analyses of their condition, the occlusion, and of the temporomandibular joint (system of mandibulomaxillary movement.)

Evaluation of prosthodontic care

In connection with epidemiological studies of tooth loss, the literature contains a variety of data on the degree of and the need for prosthodontic care. The number of teeth replaced is proposed as a measure for comparison by some authors [10, 13, 16, 17]. A comparative evaluation of the number of missing and replaced teeth in relation to age shows clear differences between young people and the middle-aged; these decrease with advancing age and thus indicate a satisfactory standard of care.

Analysis of the percentage relation of missing and replaced teeth published by various authors (Fig 4-4) indicates that territorial differences exist in the provision of dental care. More recent studies and those from rural and small town regions appear to tend towards a higher standard of care. In general, it can be assumed that 70% to 90% of missing teeth have been replaced in patients over age 60 years.

Instances of incomplete treatment and prosthetically untreated patients are included in that data, so that the true treatment needs of the group cannot be clearly characterized. Further more, nothing is said regarding the type and quality of the therapy used. The lack of objective criteria for the need for prostodontic treatment and the limits of acceptable treatment quality also leave much to be desired in the great variety of available data (Fig 4-5).

Thus, for example, *Kaden's* studies [9] of 1600 dental patients show that approximately 90% need prosthetic care. This extremely high value contrasts with the 70% to 90% rate of replaced teeth in the same age group, and can be explained only by the unacceptably poor quality of the existing treatment. This is substantiated by an earlier investigation of *Götsch*[7], that showed a need for replacement of 24% of complete dentures and 55% of removable partial dentures in 60-year-olds. Treatment needs described by *Taege* et al. [18] can be evaluated similarly.

It may be concluded, therefore, that the presently available general analyses of oral health do not indicate the true level of prosthetic care in the aged population, and that they do not reflect the real need for geriatric dental care. Specific epidemiological studies of representative groups are therefore needed.

Results of studies of geriatric dental care

Comprehensive analyses of morbidity associated with oral diseases and tooth loss and of the degree of dental care are available for the GDR from retirement homes and old age homes (Berlin, Jena, and others, 1968 to 1988). However, these are not representative of the age group as a whole, because:

- the number of persons under age 70 years is too small;

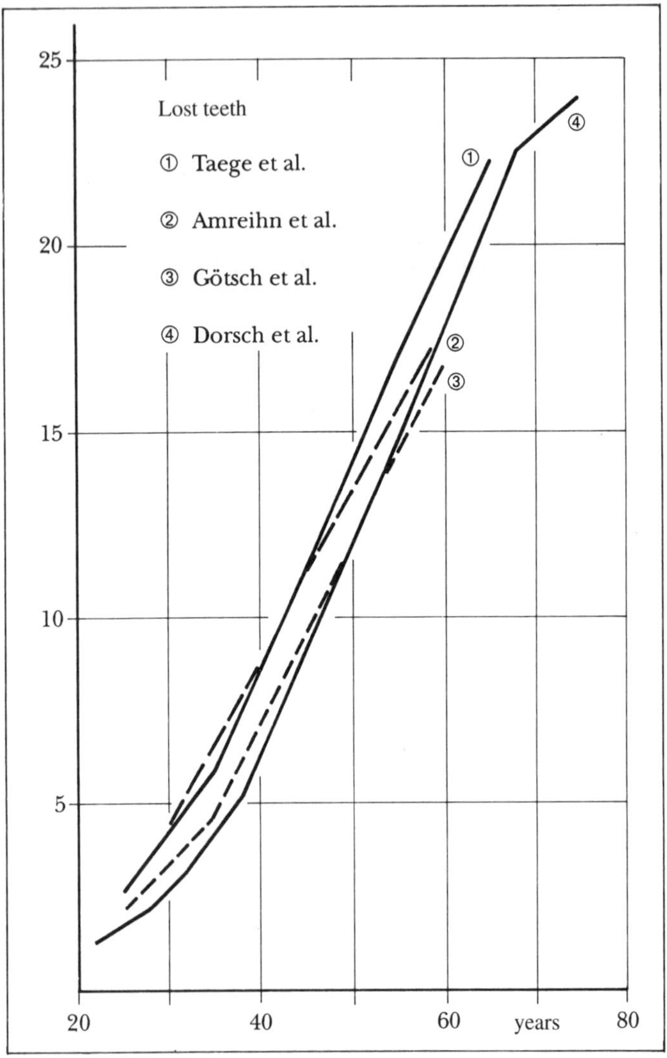

Fig. 4-4 Relation (%) of replaced and missing teeth according literature: 1 = *Knak* et al. 1975; 2 = *Sandig* 1984; 3 = *Scholz* 1986; 4 = *Lode* 1983 (see Table 4-1).

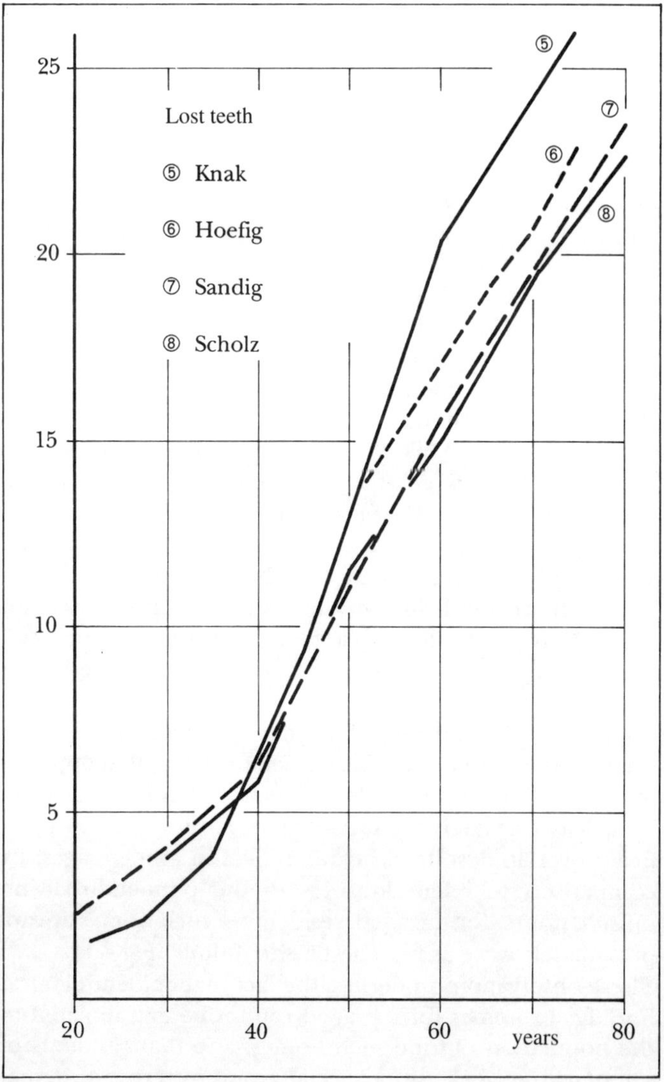

Fig. 4-5 Prosthetic requirement according different epidemiological surveys (Table 4-1).

- the number of very old persons is disproportionately large.
- the number of persons requiring nursing care is disproportionately large.

The results therefore reflect a significantly unfavourable biological and therapeutic situation, but nonetheless provide information about dental care needs of a problem, i.e. high risk, group.
Results have therefore been reported from a 10-year (1978 to 1988) study in an old age home in Erfurt [20]. The 1988 evaluation differentiated between subjects needing nursing care and other residents.
Age distribution shows a clear shift towards the very elderly groups (Fig 4-6). While 84% of all the 1978 residents were more than 70 years old, this group represented 96% of ordinary residents and 94% of nursing care residents in 1988. More than 88% of patients were older than 75 years in 1988. This trend indicates a change in the utilization of old age homes. Improved living conditions for all citzens have led the elderly to remain in single, i.e. private, residences, leaving those requiring some level of nursing care to the homes for the aged.
Analysis of the frequency of tooth loss utilizing the Eichner classification system (Table 4-2) demonstrates that approximately 85% of all probands are in class C2 and in class C3; i.e. at least one jaw is edentulous. These numbers show significant overlap despite clear differences in average ages. By comparison to edentulousness in the population living outside homes for the aged, residents of such homes are approximately twice as likely to be edentulous (Fig 4-1).
These observations underline the fact that epidemiological findings in homes for the aged cannot be extrapolated to the population outside such homes, and that residents of such facilities make up a special group in terms of dental care needs. Other data support this conclusion. When asked about their last visit to the dentist, one third of the ordinary

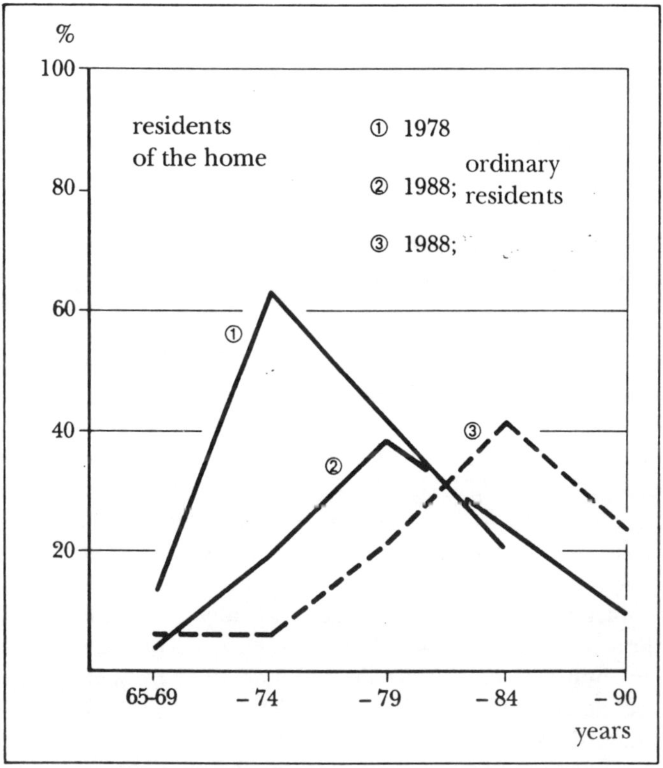

Fig. 4-6 Distribution of age for persons in nursing homes 1978 and 1988[20].

residents of old age homes and 47% of residents requiring nursing care reported that they had not received dental treatment for 15 years or longer. The time since insertion of the present dentures was correspondingly long; in 70% of the nursing care and 6.3% of the ordinary residents, the dentures had been worn for more than 10 years.

Limited function of removable prostheses was found as a consequence of the long, uncontrolled period of wear. Severe abrasion of acrylic teeth (35% to 43%) and poor

Table 4-2 Frequency of tooth loss (per cent) according to Eichner-Groups and epidemiological surveys in homes for the aged (see Fig 4-6)

Eichner groups	B3	B4	C1	C2	C3
	2.7	2.7	7.6	24.7	60.0
		5.4	9.1	20.0	65.4
	2.0	4.0	8.0	24.0	62.0

(in per cent)

seating (12% to 20%) were the most frequent flaws; in addition, nearly 25% of all prostheses required some sort of repair.

Oral mucosa changes in 29.2% of the subjects were another demonstration of unsatisfactory levels of dental care found in this study (1978). This frequency corresponds to that reported by *Welker* and *Lenz* [19], who found denture-related mucosal changes in 32.9% of old age home residents. Aetiological classification of the mucosal alterations indicated that mechanical causes (flabby ridge, hyperplasia, suction cup impressions) predominated, and their frequency was correlated with time of wear and flaws of the prostheses.

That inhabitants of these institutions make up a group with increased dental care need appears to be a justifiable conclusion, according to the results of these studies.

Proposals for further epidemiological studies

The development of a comprehensive and systematic geriatric dental care service for the entire population demands that more epidemiological data be available. Representative samples of non-institutionalized subjects aged 55 years or more should be studied to quantify:

- complete edentulousness in one or both jaws;
- partial edentulousness, differentiated according to the degree of occlusal support (number of natural teeth or Eichner groups in occlusion);
- condition of the oral hard tissue, with particular attention to abrasion, wedge-shaped defects, and root surface caries;
- condition of the periodontium and oral mucosa;
- disturbances of the temporomandibular joint (maxillo-mandibular movements);
- type of prosthesis worn and time since its insertion;
- prosthodontic care needs (type of prosthesis, repair, relining);
- treatment desires of the patient.

Bibliography

1. *Amreihn, H. and Glöckner, E.*
Zur Zweckmäßigkeit stomatologischer Morbiditätsuntersuchungen an einer Standardbevölkerung. Dtsch Stomatol 18: 830-839, (1968).

2. *Breustedt, A.*
Physiological and social factors of importance for the older edentulous patient. Int Dent J 29: 276-284, (1979).

3. *Dorsch, C. and Laetzsch, E.*
Zahnverlust und Gebißverfall beim Menschen. Dt Stomatol 23: 16-24, (1973).

4. *Eichner, K.*
Conservative and prosthetic rehabilitation procedures in the dentition of old people. Int Dent J 29: 285-297, (1979).

5. *Felgentreff, K., Höcker, M. and Schubert, R.*
Ergebnisse stomatologischer Dispensairebetreuung in Feierabend- und Pflegeheimen. Zahn-, Mund- Kieferheilkd 70: 458-464, (1982).

6. *Fröhlich, E. and Sautter, W.*
Der Gesundheitszustand des Gebisses bei unserer Bevölkerung. Dt Zahn-, Mund- Kieferheilkd 47: 675, (1959).

7. *Götsch, F. and Neubert, K.-O.*
Stomatologische Erhebungen an einer Standardbevölkerung im Kreis Sternberg. 1. Mitteilung. Dt Stomatol 23: 129-136, (1973).

8. *Hoefig, W.*
Zahnzahl älterer und alter Menschen. Dt Zahnärztl Z 29: 660-667, (1974).

9. *Kaden, E.*
Ergebnisse einer Morbiditätsuntersuchung, durchgeführt 1976 im Stadt- und Landkreis Potsdam. Stomatol DDR 30: 572-579, (1980).

10. *Knak, G. et al.*
Stomatologische Morbiditätsstudie – Berlin 1972. 4. Mitteilung. Stomatol DDR 25: 396-399, (1975).

11. *Künzel, W.*
Beitrag der Stomatologie zur Erreichung der Zielstellung "Gesundheit für alle bis zum Jahr 2000". Stomatol DDR 32: 537-541, (1983).

12. *Künzel, W., Waurick, M. and Borutta, A.*
Internationaler Vergleich des oralen Gesundheitszustandes ausgewählter Probandengruppen. Stomatol DDR 35: 81-94, (1985).

13. *Lode, D.*
Prothetisch-stomatologische Morbiditätsstudie Senftenberg 1977 und 1978. Stomatol DDR 33: 641-647, (1983).

14. *Marxkors, R.*
Aspekte zur Geriatrie in der zahnärztlichen Prothetik. Zahnärztl Praxis 37: 366-369, (1986).

15. *Rost, A.*
Lebensalter und Zahnzahl. Dt Zahnärztl Z 18: 793, (1963).

16. *Sandig, M.*
Klinische Untersuchungen über Lückengebißsituation und Art und Umfang prothetischer Therapie am Patientengut einer ambulanten stomatologischen Einrichtung der Stadt Erfurt. Med. Diss. Erfurt, 1984.

17. *Scholz, J.*
Das Lückengebiß und dessen prothetisch-therapeutische Versorgung, untersucht am Patientengut einer stomatologischen Abteilung in einem ländlichen Versorgungsbereich. Med. Diss. Erfurt, 1986.

18. *Taege, F. and Fabricius, R.*
Statistische Erhebungen über die Häufigkeit des Zahnverlustes sowie Art und Umfang der zahnärztlich-prothetischen Versorgung. Dt Zahn-, Mund- Kieferheilkd 49: 220-229, (1967).

19. *Welker, D. and Lenz, E.*
Zur Klinik und Ätiologie prothesenbedingter Veränderungen der Mundschleimheit. Stomatol DDR 25: 191-199, (1975).

20. *Wiedemann, M.*
Gerostomatologische Untersuchungen im Feierabendheim zur Ätiologie von prothesenbedingten Mundschleinhauterkrankungen. Med. Diss., Erfurt, 1978.

Chapter 5
Epidemiology of Oral Mucosal Changes from the Point of View of Geriatric Dentistry

M. Rode

Although ageing is a physiological process, it is characterized by increasing morbidity. As a consequence of long-term accumulation of very low doses of toxins, the risk of disease increases as aging proceeds.

The oral mucosa is subject to specific changes with increasing age. Such changes are caused chiefly by arteriosclerotic processes, progressive obliteration of the capillaries, and reduction in the rate of metabolism. In addition to sclerosis of the connective tissue, there is atrophy of the epithelium and bone, together with alterations in the salivary glands proceeding to the stage of xerostomia. The nerves and their end organs in the oral mucosa also may be affected by aging. Additional effects are manifested through progressive loss of sensitivity and taste acuity. The inflammatory response of tissue becomes diminished, so that ageing is accompanied by chronic atrophic processes; wound healing is slowed significantly.

The dentist must give the reactions of the oral mucosa special attention, and must be able to recognize those changes caused by aging if he is to reach appropriate conclusions. He must differentiate between the prognoses for similar oral diseases in younger and older patients, and plan treatment accordingly. Furthermore, deviations in perception must be recognized. Alterations of the oral mucosa that point to early recognition of disease may be seen during clinical examination of the oral cavity of older patients. Changes in colour and substance can be identified in the examination. In this connection, it is important and judicious that the dentist understands the epidemiology of such changes. Note that terms such as "frequent" and "rare" are inadequate to describe the incidence and prevalence of oral lesions.

Colour changes in the oral mucosa of the aged patient

White coloured lesions are the most frequent oral mucosal changes seen in the elderly.

1. Lichen planus of the oral mucosa

This dermatosis is associated with more than 50% of oral mucosal changes; in addition to whitish and keratotic efflorescences, erosions and vesicles may be seen. Lichen planus is the most common white spot oral mucosal change found in patients older than 50 years; some statistics indicate that more than 80% of lichen planus patients are over age 40[5]. Among oral pathologists, the accepted rate is 5%[8]. Preferred intraoral locations are the cheek (80%), tongue (50%), and the lips (20%)[1]. Atrophic and pemphigoid forms of lichen planus of the mucosa are frequently seen in older persons.

2. Candidiasis

a. Chronic atrophic candidiasis is caused by a yeast, *Candida albicans*. It is characterized by the presence of smooth, reddened mucosa in the region of the denture base; this form has been called stomatitis prosthetica. *Pindborg*[5] reports an occurrence rate of 10% in denture wearers over age 60; while *Ritchie*[6] claims 17%.
b. A second form is chronic hyperplastic candidiasis, the most important mycotic disease of the aged in the oral cavity. The condition is characterized by white spots which may endure for weeks or years; the spots cannot simply be wiped away. Such white spots, also described as a leukoplastic form of the disease, are most frequently seen in the retro-angular region. Differential diagnosis must include lichen planus, leukoplakia and other diseases.

3. Fordyce's disease

Heterotopic sebaceous glands are widely distributed in the oral cavity; *Bengel*[1] claims their distribution is regular. Whitish-yellow granules are seen in the lip-cheek region, a finding important in the differential diagnosis of lichen planus and leukoplakia.

4. Benign migratory glossitis (geographic tongue)

This harmless anomaly of the mucosa of the tongue is characterized by unique, greyish-white, polycyclical rings that wander over the surface during the course of the day while framing a reddened region in the tongue's centre,[1]. The condition is not infrequent (rate of occurrence is approximately 15%). Glossalgia has been reported in smokers. Attempts at treatment are not only without success; they may be harmful[3]. Benign migratory glossitis is combined with fissured tongue (lingua plicata) in about 50% of cases; the latter is a benign, congenital anomaly present in approximately 10% to 15% of the population. The deep fissures in the tongue can be a site of reduced resistance.

5. Leukoplakia

According to the WHO definition, leukoplakia is a condition characterized by white, usually sharply delineated, oral mucosal regions that cannot be rubbed off and that meets the definition of no other disease. The concept is a purely clinical one, because the definition does not rest on any histological description. Prevalence of oral leukoplakia has been examined in several nations. Occurrence in unselected populations differs. *Pindborg* reports rates of 4.9% in India, 3.6% in Hungary and 11.6% in Sweden[5]. The condition occurs predominantly in men (85:1 in India, 20:1 in Sweden). The majority of leukoplakias are found in the 40- to 70-year-old population. There is a tendency for women to develop leukoplakia somewhat later than men. Leukoplakias in the oral cavity are associated very frequently with smoking and use of tobacco, and are precancerous[9]. A precancerous lesion is defined as a morphologically altered tissue in which cancer is more probable than in an obviously normal tissue[5]. Leukoplakias – and particularly erythroplakias – must be considered to be precancerous[4]. A malignant change can be anticipated in about 6% of the flat-homogeneous form and in 24% of the dotted form.

Alterations in the substance of the oral mucosa

Some changes in the oral mucosa are characterized by increase, others by decrease in the substance of the tissue. The most important of these changes, as they are associated with aging, are closely associated with tumours.

The oral cavity cancer incidence rate can be estimated from national cancer registries. It may be seen that men have a higher oral cancer rate than women in all nations. Clear geographic differences exist in rates, however. Thus, for example, oral cancer is nearly seven times more frequent in Malta than in England (incidence in Malta: 16.9/100,000 men; in England: 2.5; in the German Democratic Republic 4.6; in Hungary 13.6; in Poland 4.0 to 8.4; in Rumania 8.7; in Slovenia 8.9, etc.). The incidence is also high in Canada (29.9) and India (19.6), while it is 9.2 in the USA (Iowa): Note, however, that it is very difficult to determine the prevalence of cancer of the oral mucosa because very few cancer registries follow the ICD-DA classification system[10].

Incidence rates of cancer in specific regions of the mouth indicate that lip cancer represents 30% of all oral cancers in Caucasians. Chronic cheilitis associated with aging must be understood to be a predisposing change of the lips. In older men, reddening of the vermillion of the lower lip, characterized by narrowing, is sometimes seen as a change. This condition is called actinic keratosis, a change that has a predisposing role in the development of carcinoma. The buccal mucosa and both oral vestibuli are locations in which oral cancer is perhaps most frequent (50% to 72% of all oral cancers)[5]. Cancer of the buccal mucosa is, above all, a disease of advanced age. In 90% of all instances, it is seen after age 40; its peak frequency arises in the 7th decade of life. Cancer of the tongue is at its highest frequency in the 6th and the 8th decades of life; similarly, all cancers of the alveolar ridge arise after age 50. The prognosis for oral cancers is poor, particularly when the diagnosis is made late. Also of epidemiological interest is perleche, a condition seen in 10% to 20% of the aged. The syndrome is multi-aetiological (infection, candidiasis, changes in the vertical dimension, etc.).

A clinically invisible, but very frequent, complication of life for the elderly is mouth burning. This is not a specific disease, but rather a not infrequent, multi-aetiological disease symptom that is particularly frequent in women of peri- and post-menopausal age and in men around age 60[3]. Eighty per cent of all women experience some burning sensation of the tongue; in more than 90% of these, the complaints are a symptom of a psychiatric disease.

All conditions associated with dry mouth can elicit a burning sensation. Some diseases and numerous drugs can cause xerostomia. Spondylosis of the cervical vertebrae can also elicit xerostomia and burning sensation of the tongue. Successful treatment of glossodynia will result only if the psychogenic factors underlying the condition are considered. Particularly in elderly patients, a burning sensation should lead to consideration of sublingual varices, which have been found in 49% of those aged more than 60 years[2].

These epidemiological facts that it is extraordinarily important to examine all elderly emphasize patients regularly, so that the presence of intraoral changes may be recognized and treated as quickly as possible.

Bibliography

1. *Bengel, W. and Veltman, G.*
Differentialdiagnostik der Mundschleimhauterkrankungen. Berlin: Quintessenz Verlag, 1986.

2. *Bouquet, J.E.*
Common oral lesions found during a mass screening examination. JADA 112:73-76, 1986.

3. *Haneke, E.*
Zungen- und Mundschleimhaut-brennen. München: Hanser Verlag, 1980.

4. *Holm-Pedersen, P. and Löe, H.*
Geriatric dentistry. Copenhagen: Munksgaard, 1986.

5. *Pindborg, J.J.*
Krebs und Vorkrebs der Mundhöhle. Berlin: Quintessenz Verlag, 1982.

6. *Ritchie, G.M.*
Die zahnärztliche Behandlung geriatrischer Patienten. Quintessenz 27:111-116, 1978.

7. *Rode, M.*
Hereditary changes of the tongue. Med Razgl 20:187-194, 1981.

8. *Rode, M.*
Lichen planus mucosae oris. Med Razgl 25:263-269, 1986.

9. *Rode, M.*
Premik, and Rode, M. The significance of the knowledge of the epidemiology of some diseases. Zdrav Vestn 52:457-459, 1982.

10. *World Health Organization.*
Application of the International Classification of Diseases to Dentistry and Stomatology. Geneva: WHO, 1978.

Chapter 6
Significance and Possibilities of Stomato-oncological Care

A. Mari

It is now an accepted view that cancer is a public disease and for effective action against it international organization is necessary. In spite of all efforts, the mortality has been increasing year by year, and what has been accepted in theory has not, in fact, been realized in practice. Considering the fact that the frequency of tumours in the oral cavity is increasing in patients *older than 50 years* – according to both the literary data and our own findings in the field of epidemiology – stomato-oncology has become a very important branch in geriatric dental research.

We are convinced that the whole body of knowledge concerning prevention, diagnostics and treatment at the disposal of the worldwide fight against cancer, used in the right way, would decrease the morbidity and mortality due to cancer.

Stomato-oncological research at the international level is directed by the WHO and UICC. In Hungary the programme of cancer prevention is organized according to that recomended by the WHO (Expert Committee on Early Detection of Cancer), the main points of which are: prevention; early recognition; diagnosis; treatment; follow-up; after-care; rehabilitation.

In prevention, each carcinogenic factor (physical, chemical, endogenic factors, viruses, etc.) which may have a carcinogenic role according to experiments on laboratory animals and epidemiological findings must be eliminated. In the organization dealing with the task of prevention, it is important that dental examinations should also become an oncological screening test and that suspected cancerous cases should be admitted to the right institute as soon as possible. Taken together, lung and dental screening would increase the number of reported cases. Lectures for the general public as well as special ones for doctors and dentists should be regularly given at a level which would convince the audience of the great importance of prevention and the possibility of avoiding its development.

There are two methods of prevention: one is individual and the other is performed by the state. In individual prevention, people with sufficient knowledge for self-examination may discover a precancerous symptom. As for prevention by the state, the conviction is spreading world wide that the fight against cancer is a task for the community, that is for the state. This has also achieved international importance, taking into account agreements between states and the situation in the state of each signatory concerning its report on the causes, natures, spread and treatment. The basic factors in stomato-oncological care, both in Hungary and abroad, are the epidemiological examinations. However, in order to be able to take part in this international movement, we need to use a language understood by all participants and devise an oncological questionnaire for computerization as a sine qua non. The epidemiological examinations should answer the following questions:

- Frequency of stomato-oncological diseases and planning possible demand for their treatment (instrumentation and staff).

- What factors play a role in the frequency and distribution of stomato-oncological disease.

- What factors contribute to the decision regarding the type of treatment necessary (laboratory findings at tissue examination, TNM system, localization).
- What results may be achieved by health education for the population in the field of oncology (newspapers, radio, TV) and what improvement may be expected in the fight against cancer.
- To reach the above-mentioned aims, what facilities and what number of doctors and ancillary medical personnel would be necessary.
- Decide that for the success of the programme, basic education and also refresher courses would be necessary.
- Deciding the possible suitability of medical institutes for coping with the work of prevention, treatment and follow-up, in short, all the high level performance of care, and plan their material needs for successful function.
- On the basis of collected data, ranking these institutes in order to maximise the utilization of the financial contribution of the state towards boosting the results of stomato-oncological care.
- The stomato-oncological work performed in these institutes should be regularly supervised and – when necessary – new measures should be taken if changes make it necessary.

The main task of screening should be *early recognition,* that is great efforts should be made to discover a precancerous stage when virtually no definite symptoms are present (preclinical stage). It is important that the patient, with the help of previous health education, should recognize the early danger signals (colour change in the mucous membrane, overgrowth of tissues, non healing wounds, ulcers, scabs, bleeding etc.).

The depressing Hungarian and foreign statistical data show that even today it is usually a long time after the appearance of the first symptoms before the patient goes to his doctor and appropriate treatment can be started; and this sad situation is hindering the necessary cooperation between doctor and patient that is one of the most important factors for achieving good results.

The prognosis of oral carcinoma is much better when an *early diagnosis* can be made. An early diagnosis is not difficult, because the oral cavity is easy to examine by sight and precancerous lesions and other tumour-causing diseases are not difficult to spot. As with gynaecological screening, an almost ideal situation would be, if at the first medical observation, interview of the patient, along with clinical examination and cytological sample, would convince him or her of the necessity to report for treatment and to be taken into special care. For the final diagnosis, biopsy should be performed only in an institute or stomato- oncological centre where adequate facilities are available. Naturally, all other necessary equipment for up-to-date diagnostics (X-ray apparatus, laboratory, etc.) should be at the disposal of the medical staff. From the point of view of prevention, most important is the expertise which is the basis of making the clinical diagnosis. That is why it is so very important for the dentist to be able to recognize precancerous lesions and other possible disorders from a good knowledge of differential diagnostics. Recently, cancer research has turned its attention towards the study of precarcinomas, which offers effective possibilities for prevention. The responsibility is considerable for the doctor who has seen the patient for the first time, for a not entirely precise initial diagnosis is an error easier to overcome than treatment which is not adequate, and this frequently happens. Such harmful practice may frustrate any future effort to save the patient. That is why strict supervision is so necessary, of both the patient and the inexperienced doctor, to increase the effect of modern stomato-oncology.

Complex treatment has in principle not changed as far as tumours in the oral cavity are concerned, yet in each institute where oncological treatment has been practised for some time, certain dominant methods have been developed and preferences have been formed. Each method has its own limitations, to which a number of influencing factors must be added (localization, laboratory cytological findings, X-ray sensitivity, nearness of bone, age of patient, etc.). It has been acknowledged worldwide that a plan for oncological treatment needs the recommendation of a group containing a surgeon, X-ray specialist, chemotherapist, oncologist and pathologist with equal weights of opinions. Alas, this idealistic plan has not become accepted in practice, and even now it is difficult to change the beliefs both of the layman and of many doctors that, apart from surgical treatment, other newer methods can be effectively applied in the treatment of tumours, especially in elderly patients when their advantages are apparent. Even in tumour surgery ultraradical methods (mutilations, deformations) seem to be decreasing and limited surgery is becoming more popular. In cases where a larger facial defect seems to be inevitable, the surgeon must make the greatest effort to restore it by plastic surgery at the same time that the tumour is eradicated. If plastic surgery would not produce acceptable results, the defect must be referred to the prosthetician for supplementation. That is why each oncological centre needs a well equipped unit and an expert staff with the necessary training in this branch of prosthetics. Nowadays in the treatment of oral tumours irradiation is unavoidable (interstitial therapy, devices functioning on million volt sources of irradiation, afterloading device, etc.).

Considering that modern surgical treatment (including plastic surgery), irradiation and chemotherapy place an extraordinary financial burden on every institute, it would appear sensible that a limited number of well equipped stomato-oncological centres should be set up. The treatment of oncological patients aims not only to cure them or keep them alive for some time longer, but while alive, they should have a tolerable life. Unfortunately, the issue of institutional care of incurable cases has not yet been solved. Apart from the treatment of oncological diseases, the oncological centre should cope with follow-up and after-care of their patients.

In oncological care the results should not be judged only on treatment efficacy at the first stage but also on the prevention of recurrences, metastases, or at least early discovery and adequate treatment. Practice shows the importance of the frequency of post-therapy care, i.e. the creation of an outpatient department for stomato- oncological care to check the condition of treated patients at regular intervals. The treatment of recurrences and metastases is usually performed on the same principles as the primary treatment, and for this reason repeated treatments must be performed at the same stomato-oncological centre.

Apart from physical rehabilitation, a stomato-oncological patient needs both moral and spiritual rehabilitation too. It is also necessary in incurable cases, when the patient is admitted into an institute for permanent care, that he or she should not feel absolute hopelessness towards the last tragic period leading to their death, which should be made as dignified as possible.

We think that there is an urgent need to invite practising psychologists into the oncological organization, who, together with experts in oncological care, would help the majority of mostly elderly patients to overcome their fear of cancer (carcinophobia) and other complicated psychological troubles by alleviating them as far as possible.

There is no branch of medicine where integration and centralization can have such a definitive role as in oncology. Efforts should be made worldwide to equip oncological centres – including those in Hungary at the level of present day medical science in oncology, with the target of adequate and constant funding to enable them to undertake all forms of treatment, along with the adaptation of new and proven methods and organization of their own research.

Bibliography

1. *Bánoczy, J.*
Die Früherkennung der Mundhöhlenkarzime. Zahnärztekalender S. 257-265, 1963.

2. *Bánoczy, J., Radnei, I. and Reményi, I.*
Methodological experiences based on stomato-oncological examinations made in the population of Dunakeszi and Felsógöd. Fogorv Szle 62:118-122, 1969.

3. *Bruszt, P.*
Stomato-oncological screening examinations in the region of Baja and Bácsalmás. Magyar Onkol 6:28-33, 1962.

4. *Pindborg, J.J.*
Conference on epidemiology of oral cancer and precancerous lesions. Report of Proceedings. Int Dent J 18:626-630, 1968.

5. *Corso, P.F.*
Rehabilitation of patients with oral cancer. Surg Clin N Am 53:607-624, 1969.

6. *Einhorn, I. and Wersäll, I.*
Incidence of oral carcinoma in patients with leukoplakia of the oral mucosa. Cancer 20:2189-2193, 1967.

7. *Fasske, E. et al.*
Die Früherkennung des Carcinoms in der Mundhöhle. Dtsch Zahnärztl Z 14:251-253, 1959.

8. *Kimmel, K.*
Dentist against cancer. Diagnosis, prevention and therapy of oral carcinoma. Quintessenz 19:35-37, 1968.

9. *Pindborg, J.J.*
Oral cancer and precancer as diseases of aged. Commun Dent Oral Epidemiol 6:300-307, 1978.

10. *Pindborg, J.J.*
Epidemiological studies of oral cancer. Int Dent J 27:172-178, 1977.

11. *Sallay, K.*
Szájbetegségek (Oral Diseases) pp 199-203. Budapest: Medicina 1984.

12. *Vándor, F.*
Diagnosis and therapy of tumors of the oral cavity, pharynx and upper respiratory system. Budapest: Thesis, 1969.

13. *WHO.*
Collaborating Centre for oral precancerous lesions. Definition of leukoplakia and related lesions. An aid to studies on oral precancer. Oral Surg 46:518-539, 1978.

Part III Psychosocial Aspects

Chapter 7
Psychosocial Problems in Geriatric Dental Care from the Point of View of the Dentist

M. Höcker

Due to the aim of preserving the physical, psychical and social well-being of the elderly and thus their physical powers, by means of complex care, quantitatively and especially qualitatively new problems also arise in the field of stomatology [1, 2, 5-7, 9-11]. Insufficient dental care not only has immediate consequences in the sense of faster destruction of the oral structures, but also drastic effects on physical and psychical powers, particularly of aged persons. Attention must be paid both to digestive disorders caused by impaired masticatory capacity resulting in deficit malnutrition, as well as to psychological aspects. It must be presumed that functional losses in the orofacial region have negative effects on the self-assessment of aged persons and their social integration, and can involve psychical alterations in the sense of genuine illness (e.g. psychogenous denture incompatibility).

On the other hand, masticatory ability and the absence of discomfort add greatly to a positive attitude towards life and to ego and social interaction, thus constituting the basis for

the well-being of the elderly. Moreover, their attitude concerning their demands for dental care is decided to a high degree by psychosocial factors. Therefore, knowledge of this causal relationship is of great importance for the strategy of caring for the different groups of aged citizens as well as to successful rehabilitation in individual cases.
Therefore, local and especially general factors must be considered as variables in the field of dental care for aged citizens [8].

Local factors

- number and functional capacity of the natural dentition
- quality of restoratory and rehabilitatory measures
- functional deficits or their compensation, respectively
- locally caused psychological alterations
- hygiene of mouth and dental plate
- metaphylaxis

General factors

- general state of health
- conditions of living
- sensorial-perceptive capacities
- manual capacities
- state of attendance characterized by approachability and acceptance, consciousness of oral health, personal experience and individual preferences
- economic status dependent upon the existing welfare system

The purpose of the following is, therefore, to highlight and analyse psychosocial problems with reference to findings in literature, complemented by results of personal tests. To begin with, it must be stated that the image which elderly patients have of their dentist has advanced from the "academi-

Table 7-1 Statements on own dentist (Höcker 1983) (n = 306, mean age = 66.8 years)

Characteristic	%
Only interested in the teeth	44.8
Inquires also about general problems	18.9
Possesses empathy	13.0
No good experience	6.5
No opinion	16.8

cal mechanic" to the specialized physician, from whom the elderly derive corresponding expectations as to care and welfare on the part of the dentist.

Tests with students of a university for students of advanced years, however, showed that approximately 45% were of the opinion that dentists are only concerned with teeth (Table 7-1).

The results demonstrate clearly that the dentist pays too little consideration to the patients'personality and living conditions.

Considering the general factors of the structure of dental care conditions, communication between dentist and patient takes a key position.

With increasing age, a trustful relationship between dentist and patient becomes more vital than the therapy itself in the strictest sense and must be considered an integral part of diagnostics and of the entire care. In this connection, attention must be paid to the already considerable interindividual variation, which increases with advancing years. Moreover, it must be taken into consideration, that, because of an essentially higher educational level and of a different lifestyle, the level of demands that future generation of pensioners will have will rise steadily.

In 2005, for instance, the proportion of graduate old-age pensioners in the GDR will increase by three times and of those pensioners with a technical training by four times.

Table 7-2 Efficiency of overdentures – objective

Funcitonal degree	Upper jaw n	Upper jaw %	Lower jaw n	Lower jaw %
Sufficient	138	65.4	98	70.0
Insufficient	73	34.6	42	30.0

Thus, the quality of the dentist-patient relationship is directly connected with older people's need for security, and has great influence on compliance and the patients'satisfaction with the therapeutic effect. Not least is a standard of acceptance and attendance, which is an essential criterion for the use of dental care.

This attitude of elderly people as to their demands for attendance is of decisive importance in the light of the caring strategy. As a general principle, it must be presumed that the objective need for care is distinctly greater than the demands made by the patients, and that subjective contentment, even with obvious objective defectiveness of dentures or of the remaining teeth and the symptom-free state going with increasing indolence do not induce the patients to demand attendance (Tables 7-2, 7-3).

Moreover, the attitude to demands for attendance is influenced, positively or negatively, by the following factors:

- Number of remaining teeth – old patients who still possess their own teeth tend to consult a dentist more readily, than toothless ones, though occurring trouble is the most important reason. In the light of the change in morbidity (caries decline) which is to be expected, an increasing demand for attendance has to be taken into account. Patients provided with complete dentures, on the other hand, when the adaptation has been performed, usually demand attendance only when experiencing serious discomfort. Not least by reason of limited information from

Table 7-3 Efficiency of overdentures – subjective

Functional degree	Upper jaw n	Upper jaw %	Lower jaw n	Lower jaw %
Sufficient	177	83.9	96	68.6
Insufficient	34	16.1	44	31.4

the dentist, they are of the opinion that with their »third dentition«, they have no more need of dental care.

- Age according to the calendar or the biological age, respectively. It must be presumed that with advancing years, contacts with the dentist become more and more rare; at present, the interval may frequently be up to 10 years. On the other hand, when adequately motivated, aged persons who remained biologically young may develop earnest demands for dental care, which definitely must be met.
- Sex . Sex also has significance as to demands for attendance. Women's attitude, on the whole, is more positive. In this context it must be emphasized that, because of the greater expectation of life, the percentage of women is steadily increasing with advancing years, with two out of three living beyond the 70th year of age.
  Furthermore, it has to be taken into consideration that men tend to overestimate their state of health, while women tend to underestimate it.
- General state of health and mobility. Limited ability to walk and malaise following various general ailments (polypathy) have a negative influence on the demand for dental care. Often, six to eight diseases with their respective physical and psychological impairments are evident in aged citizens. About 20% of the elderly in the widest sense can be classified as needing medical care and 6% to 8% as needing nursing [3].
- Psychological state. With regard to the attitude towards dental care, psychological alterations which result from

the pain of general systemic illness, but are caused much more by growing isolation, and therefore from absent social interaction (transition to the old age pensioner state, retiring from professional activity, decrease of self-esteem, loss of family members, loneliness, giving up of own flat with entrance into a home for aged people) are of great importance and lead to relative indifference towards dental care.

On the other hand, the maintenance of social contacts (group effect) may also induce a positive behaviour pattern.

– Degree and level of medical care within the residential area. Under the aspect of increasing disability, easy access to stomatological care and the subsequent acceptance of this attendance are very important for aged subjects. It is evident that, at present, there exist barriers in the attitude of dentists as well as of aged patients (Tables 7-4 and 7-5).

  Aged patients require special consulting hours and more sensitivity in caring on the part of the dentist, and complain of lack of time, lack of interest, unfriendly treatment and lack of understanding. Not least, inappropriate behaviour patterns on the part of dentists are evident, which result from ignorance about the problems of the elderly and have a negative influence on aged persons' willingness to accept dental care.

  In this connection, inquiries made of dental students effectively illustrated the poor psychological training they received in the course of their studies (Tables 7-6 and 7-7).

– Level of information. At present, most aged persons lack information on the importance of efficient oral and denture hygiene and on the necessity of a regular health check, even with their third dentures.

  This lack of information must be considered a factor of sociogenic risk, and must be attributed to the fact that the majority of the dentists do not comply with the strict

Table 7-4 Critiscism of dental attendance (n = 146)

Characteristic	n	%
No criticism	80	54.6
No family dentist	11	7.5
Impersonal treatment	19	13.0
Long waiting periods	35	24.0
Dentist has too little time	16	11.0
Barriers of communication	3	2.1

Table 7-5 Expectations as to the dentist (n = 146)

Characteristic	n	%
Best attendance	117	80.1
Empathy	4	2.7
Special consulting hours	19	13.0
Exact information	107	73.3
Consideration of private wishes	14	9.6
Understanding and care	27	8.5
No expectations	9	6.2
Other answers	4	2.7

(several answers were possible)

demand for information and motivating influence, though persistently desired by aged patients (Table 7-7).

Thus, it may be stated on the one hand, in view of efficient stomatological care for citizens of advanced age and old people clinical-technical perfection constitutes an absolute prerequisite, and on the other hand, the consideration of general factors, like the general state of health, the social environment, previous experience in the field of stomatological attendance, the dentist's motivation to treat aged patients, and the consideration of aged patients' expectations

Table 7-6 Necessity of fundamental psychological knowledge (n = 191)

Characteristic	%
Absolutely necessary	55.5
Turn up in the course of professional activity	35.6
No evaluation possible	8.9

Table 7-7 Psychological training during studies (n = 199)

Characteristic	%
Amplification necessary	56.2
Insufficient	22.8
Sufficient	17.5
No evaluation possible	3.5

are of decisive importance in individual therapeutic success and particularly to an organized mode of care for this group.

The following consequences result:

1. In the field of research it is necessary to obtain by means of representative studies within individual groups (pre-pensioner age, handicapped and non-handicapped elderly) obligatory statements as to the identified psychosocial problems.
2. Based on these perceptions, there follows the necessity to enable stomatologists and their fellow-workers in a process of education, continued professional training and development, to take care of aged citizens.
3. Finally, there arises the demand for putting into practice knowledge and experience in the process of dental care, using them as the basis for the concept of dental care and therapeutic success.

Bibliography

1. *Bates, J.F., Adams, D. and Stafford G.D.*
   Zahnärztliche Behandlung älterer Patienten. Berlin: Quintessenz Verlag, 1986.

2. *Breustedt, A.*
   Stomatologische Betreuung im höheren Lebensalter. Leipzig: Barth Verlag, 1978.

3. *Eitner, S.*
   Aktivität im Alter als Ziel von Vorbereitung auf das Alter und komplexer Betreuung im Alter, pp 16-27 In Gerontologie – Heute, Schriftenreihe der Gesellschaft Gerontologie der DDR und des Forschungsprojektes Gerontologie der DDR. Berlin, vol. 14, 1979.

4. *Höcker, M.*
   Zahnärztliche Aspekte bei der Vorbereitung auf ein gesundes Alter. Z. Gerontol 16: 553-57, 1983.

5. *Höcker, M.*
   Vergleichende stomatologische Erhebungen zur oralen Gesundheit in den verschiedenen Lebensaltern, Med. Diss. B. Berlin, 1983.

6. *Imfeld, Th.*
   Alterszahnmedizin – Herausforderung der Zukunft. Swiss Dent 6: 21-33, 1985.

7. *Körber, E. (ed)*
   Die zahnärztlich-prothetische Versorgung des älteren Menschen. München: C. Hanser Verlag, 1978.

8. *Kiyak, H.A. and Benett, J.*
   In B.D. Ingersoll Psychologische Aspekte der zahnärztlichen Betreuung. Berlin: Quintessenz Verlag pp 129-145, 1987.

9. *Künzel, W.*
   International Collaborative Study of Dental Manpower Systems – Anliegen und Ziele. Stomatol DDR 35: 57-62, 1985.

10. *Künzel, W.*
    Die Forschung als Grundlage stomatologischer Betreuungsstrategie. pp 177-195 – in: Medizin und Gesellschaft 31 VEB. Berlin: Verlag Volk und Gesundheit, 1987.

11. *Sauerwein, E. (ed)*
    Alterszahnheilkunde, 2nd edition. Stuttgart: Thieme Verlag, 1983.

Chapter 8
Psychosocial Problems in Geriatric Dental Care from the Point of View of the Psychologist

J. Šopek and V. Šícha

The basic task of a health care policy in a socialist society is to provide people from all walks of life with adequate preventive and health care.

A significant task in this respect is the health and social care of older and elderly citizens. This fact is illustrated in the Czechoslovak Socialist Republic by the following statistics.

In 1985 there were 15.5 million people living in the Czechoslovak Socialist Republic. Of these, 1.7 million (i.e. 11.1%) were older then 65 and 314,000 older than 80 years (i.e. 2.1%). The demographic forecast predicts that by the end of the year 1990 the number of citizens over 65 years of age will exceed 2 million (i.e. 12.5% of the population) and the number of citizens over 80 years of age will exceed 0.4 million (about 2.5% of the population). Interestingly, the number of people over 65 in the city of Brno already exceeds 13% (over 50,000 out of 386,000 people).

By the end of the year 2000 the proportion of old people in the population of the Czechoslovak Socialist Republic will increase still further and the number of citizens over 65 will exceed 15%. The index of the probable age expectancy of those who are now reaching 60 is clearly increasing; it is necessary to think of these people as living for another 20 years or so. In connection with this development, the tasks of geriatric care, which are reflected in every branch of medicine, are growing. The tasks of dentistry are clearly influenced by the problems connected with the solution to the process of human ageing.

It is necessary to make a basic re-evaluation of the traditional concept of old age as a negative, unproductive and useless period of life, that old people are of little use. We must face the real danger that the prolongation of life may mean, for a large group of the population, a sort of survival or poor existence on the edge of a society of young and productive people. Supporting senior citizens, like child care, is an important factor in the standard of living in every society. Our interest in serving the older generation is shown by the long-term universal social and health programme, laid down in the conclusions of the Party congresses and other binding documents. But at the same time, it is clear that care for old people is determined by progress in creating material and social values as a prerequisite for positive steps.

In addition to general health reasons, there are other significant reasons for the increasing importance of dental care of the older generation:

1. The relationship between the condition of the dentition and chewing apparatus on the one hand and problems with digestion and nutrition on the other hand; these must be thought of in terms of their mutual inter-relationships, consequences and circumstances – both health and social, and ultimately also economic.
2. The problems of the place of old people in society, their social activities, subjective problems and complaints, experience, self evaluation and self reflection are not only significant factors influencing the quality of their life and their contentment (the personal and social importance of the facial region) but also represent a prerequisite for

their continuing social contribution, usefulness and independence.

The need for the dental care of old people is underlined by objective and subjective aspects. Yet, practical geriatric dentistry in the Czechoslovak Socialist Republic is being developed slowly and inadequately. There are several *reasons for this unsatisfactory state*:

1. Old people lose strength and resistance and polymorbidity appears in all aspects relating to health. The functional state of the tissues of an old person is qualitatively different, as a rule poorer. This makes specific demands on the choice of treatment, on the technique and extent of interventions, on materials and applied medication.
2. The social activity of old people decreases in comparison with the productive years; old people are less active in arranging their examination, treatment and therapy. Nor are the efforts of dentists in inviting old people to their consulting rooms or visiting them welcomed with interest and gratitude. Old people often respond with mistrust and have a feeling of being pushed into something.
3. The social standing, prestige, standard of living and economic situation of old people are usually lower.
4. Generally speaking, the quality of life decreases in old age. The dentition problems of old people are only a portion of their other problems, difficulties and sense of insecurity. Although they attend their local doctor quite often (approximately 6 to 10 times a year), they very seldom go to the dentist. Their dentition problems do not seem to them to be as urgent as some of their other health problems.
5. With growing age the ability to create new dynamic stereotypes worsens, as does adaptibility. This is negatively manifested, for example, in a poorer attitude to dentures.
6. There is a shift in the mental attitude of old people; negative qualities, previously compensated for, now emerge

in a form difficult to accept. Old people are suspicious, vulnerable and have a tendency towards negative views of themselves in retrospect and resignation – all this is easily reinforced by the reactions of their surroundings. In thought processes, we can often find fixations and distorted thinking. The sense of hearing and memory get worse. Communication with other people is rather difficult. Orientation, expecially in unknown and unfamiliar situations, becomes a problem.

7. The health and social services are not sufficient to keep pace with the growing proportion of old people in our population. The existing shortcomings of our health care system also affect dentistry, and are more clearly evident in connection with older citizens. Dental health services for old people are limited by a shortage of some technical aids, appliances, health materials and drugs.
   When a selection is made as to who will be provided with limited, difficult or expensive services, the old are usually neglected.
8. For the dentist, cooperation with old people is usually more difficult and takes longer, demanding more time, activity and patience. To work with an old person is less rewarding, not only from the medical viewpoint but also socially and sometimes materially as well.

For progress in the objective concrete dental care of old people, these negative influences form an unfavourable situation. We hope, however, that the new Commission for Gerostomatology, established in Autumn 1986 under Dr MUDr A. Dapeci, CSc, within the Stomatological Society of the J.E. Purkyně Czech. Medical Society, will gradually solve these problems.
For the immediate future, we consider the following targets of prime importance in the dental care of old people:

1. To deepen our knowledge of the health and especially dental needs of our older generation.
2. To devote continuous attention to geriatric dental re-

search and other means of increasing our knowledge of geriatric dentistry. It is necessary to work from an interdisciplinary approach and a thorough understanding of the biopsychosocial correlations.

3. To publicize geriatric dental information through the activities of the professional societies and in the professional journals and publications.
4. To ensure that the biopsychosocial and more specifically working and technical problems of geriatric dentistry are better represented in the pregraduate and specialized preparation of dentists.
5. To consider the participation of psychologists in the research, teaching and practical tasks of geriatric dentistry.
6. In the legislative sphere, to waive the extra fees for work on fixed protheses (in Czechoslovakia this is a service which must be paid for partially by the patient). This is an anachronism that is in contradiction to the principle of free socialist health care. A positive impact can be expected, especially in the prosthetic care of old people. Presently, the extra fee for fixed protheses, even though precious metals are not used, can be such a financial burden for the old that they refuse treatment.
7. Amendments to the Programme for the Field of Stomatology are currently being worked out. It is expected that the duty to provide active dental care for our older and chronically ill citizens, regardless of whether they are living in families, old people's homes or hospitals for old and chronically ill people, will be set out and institutionalized therein.
8. Furthermore, in the interest of better dental care for older citizens it is necessary to work out forms of cooperation between local dentists and local general practitioners or geriatric nurses working in the neighbourhoods. It is no less important to deepen the organizational follow-up and cooperation between the dental surgery and specialists in the appropriate local health area (internal specialists, neurologists etc.).

Bibliography

1. *Dapeci, A., Houzar, I., Smékal, M., Sopek, I. and Sigmund I.*
Celkové animatelné náhrady u pacientu vyssich vekových skupin. Csl stomatol 83:143-149, 1983.

2. *Donek, E. and Kemr, M.*
Stári a psychika. Prakt Lék 68:49-51, 1988.

3. *Hosek, K. and Kemr, M.*
Nekteré sociálne psychologické a zdravotni charakteristiky starých lidi v populaci okresu UH. Csl Psychiatrie 83:251-257, 1987.

4. *Krivohlavý, J.*
Sociálni komunikace se starými lidmi. Zdrav Pracovnice 4:215-221, 1987.

5. *Idvecke, E.*
Uvod do gerontopedagogiky. Praha: OSI MS, 1979.

6. *Malická, L.*
Zpusob zivota v duchodovém veku. Sociol Cas 5:487-500, 1987.

7. *Smutná, R.*
Zdravotni a socialni stav obcanu vyssiho veku. Prag: Zpravy VUPs, 1987.

8. Statistická rocenka CSSR 1987. Prag: SNTL-Verlag, 1988.

9. *Sopek, J. and Sicha, V.*
Psychologická hlediska stomatologické péce o starou generaci. Prakt Zubni lék 30:166-171. 1982.

Part IV Regional Epidemiological Data

Chapter 9
Geriatric Dental Care in Prague

V. Mareš

We carried out an epidemiological study on a group of 735 old and elderly subjects, living in geriatric establishments in three Prague districts. We were investigating their dentition and oral tissue state, especially the number of edentulous patients, number of natural teeth, demands for treatment, mode and extent of dental treatment and its specialities. We have found out that the most urgent need is for treatment in dental prosthetics, especially in making removeable dentures followed by conservative dentistry and oral surgery. We have also found out that in old persons demands for treatment are much lower than treatment needs. It is therefore necessary to improve health education and access to dentists.

On the basis of our experience and epidemiological research we have derived conclusions for realization in practice. We recommend the setting up of one or more geriatric dentistry centres in each Prague district, with an adequate number of nurses. The chief physician of such an establishment will be responsible for control of geriatric dental care in all establishments in the respective district. Further, we recommend the setting up, according to resources, of individual dental workplaces in all major geriatric establishments, to extend geriatric dental education in pre- and postgraduate education with stress on psychological and ethical aspects.

When planning development of geriatric dental care and its implementation we must start with the prognoses of demographic structure of inhabitants and changes in the mode of geriatric dentistry care in the near future.

The awaited changes will involve extending of geriatric dental care, prosthetics treatment, and conservative and parodontological treatment for the increasing number of permanent teeth. Important also will be deepening of prevention in geriatric dentistry.

Material and methods

For an epidemiological study of the needs of geriatric dental treatment and its organization, we consider it important to know the number of people in each age category.

We do not consider classification by nurses very suitable in this case because it covers large age groups (15 years) in individual categories and there are big differences between individuals in need of treatment and in changes in their oral tissues.

In our study for persons over 60 we therefore use four categories, each one with an age bracket of 10 years.

For the entire Prague population of 1,197,500 persons we have 209,000 persons over 60. They can be divided into four categories according to Table 9.1.

We began to examine patients in geriatric establishments in three Prague districts – Prague 4, 8 and 10. The group represents 735 persons (583 women, 152 men). We know that such a group does not represent all the elderly people in Prague, but they are persons who generally have the same access to treatment.

Examination was made with mirror and tube in daylight or dental lights which were available in geriatric establishments

Table 9-1

Age group	Number of persons	Men	Women
60 to 69	99,900	44,870 45%	54,830 55%
70 to 79	78,100	33,000 42%	45,100 58%
80 to 89	25,100	8,100 32,8%	17,000 67,2%
90	6,050		not stated

in the respective districts. There were subjects aged 60 to 99 in the group.

We investigated age and sex of the patients, number of visits to the dentist in 1986, edentulousness of both jaws, dentures, and number of teeth in both dental bows. Further, we asked about treatment in 1986 – surgical treatment, conservative treatment, periodontological treatment, making dentures and their repairs. We also observed diseases of the oral mucous membrane which required treatment. These included leukoplakia, glossodynia, dry mouth and smooth tongue. From the point of view of treatment we also observed the occurrence of cheilosis praecanceromatosa and carcinoma.

In general medical examination we noted diabetus mellitus, hypertension, cardiac diseases and IM.

With regard to the methodology itself, we emphasize that each epidemiological study, either Czechoslovakian or from abroad, and each partial investigation has different methodology and fixed parameters.

To compare different studies it would be appropriate to find common methods for all studies and partial investigations in geriatric dentistry.

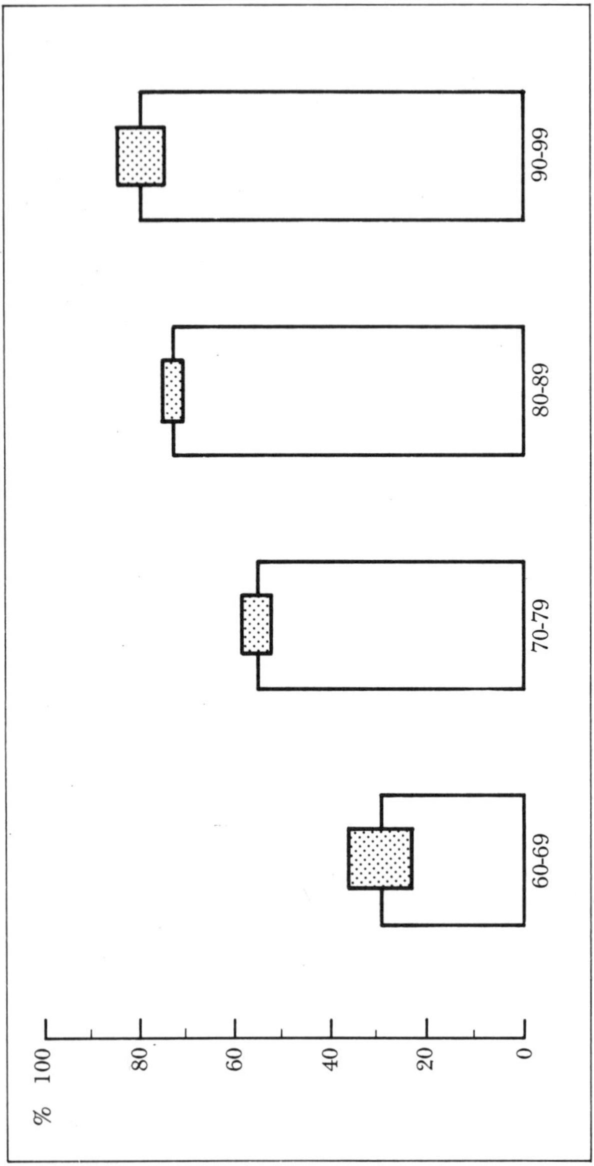

Fig. 9-1 Percentage of edentulous in different age groups.

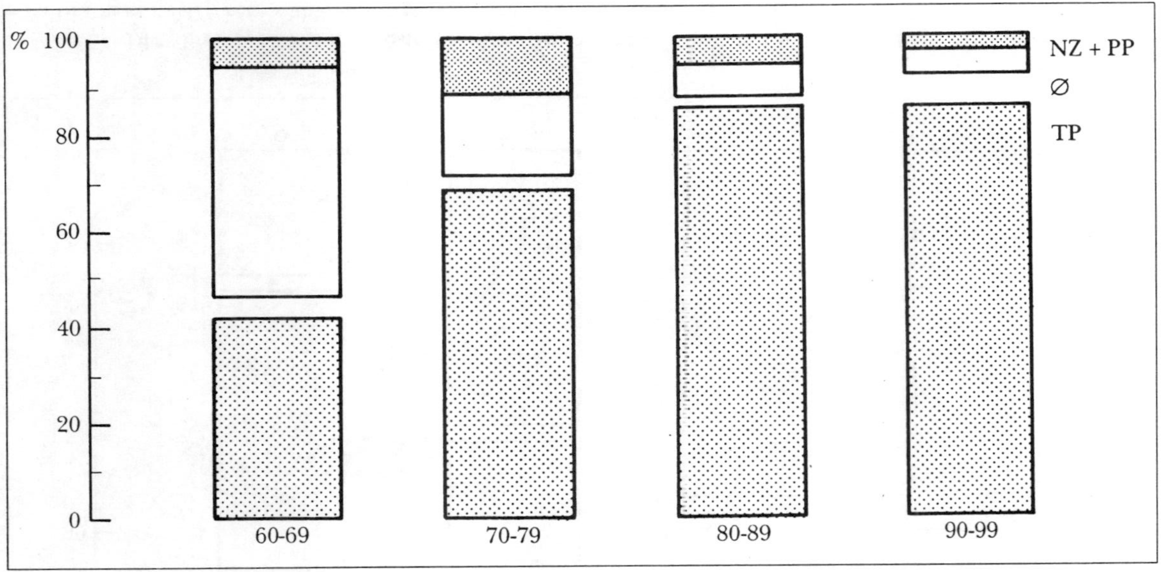

Fig. 9-2 a Distribution of edentulousness and percentage of persons with removable dentures, upper jaw; NT = natural teeth, RE = removable denture, TD = total denture and ª = edentulousness.

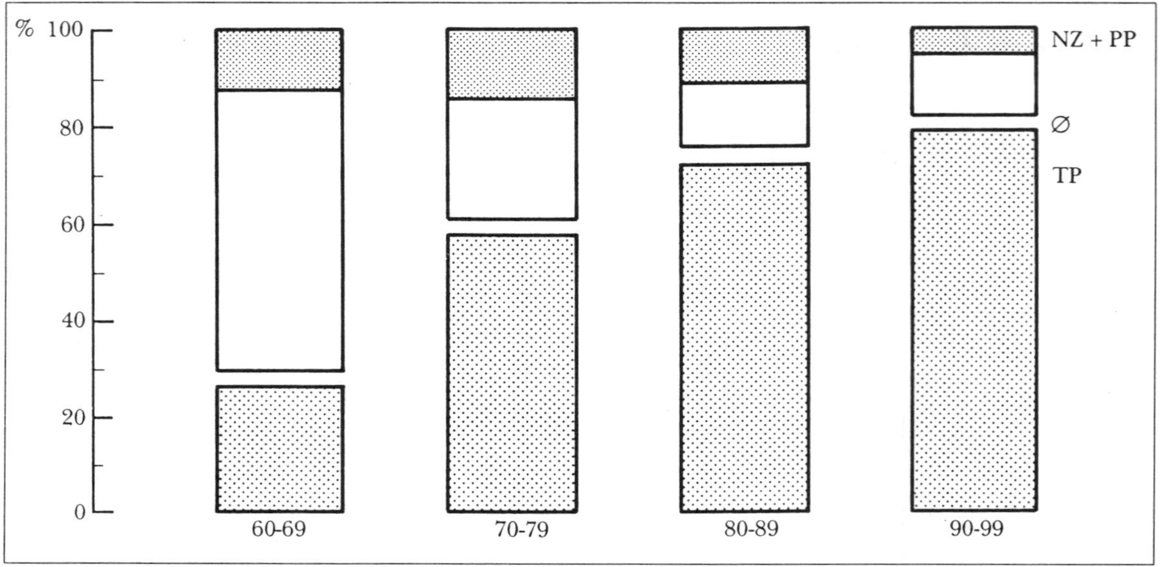

Fig. 9-2 b Distribution of edentulousness and percentage of persons with removable dentures, upper jaw; NT = natural teeth, RE = removable denture, TD = total denture and [a] = edentulousness.

Results and documentation

The documentation of all 735 persons contains serial number, first letter of name, date of birth and sex. Then we presented all the parameters mentioned in methodology. The results of our work are presented in the form of nine graphs, with relevant comments.

Discussion

There are many papers on geriatric dentistry and its problems. The practical needs of dental care for older people are important epidemiological studies which show clearly the state of the oral cavity and dentition in old people and at the same time show the necessity of dental care. Unfortunately, individual groups are very different as far as methodology is concerned. That is why it is very difficult, nearly impossible, to compare the results. This is certainly true also for our work and patient group, which was studied with regard to the needs of basic dental treatment for people living in geriatric establishments.

Unification of the system of recording the data concerning the state of the oral cavity is also one of the main tasks of the WHO and FDI programme "Health for All by year 2000" (WHO, 1983).

According to this outline we can divide Prague districts into three groups. In the first one we can include Prague 1, 2, 3 and 7 with the lowest number of persons over 60. In the second one, Prague 5, 6, 8, 9 and 10 with average numbers of persons over 60. The third group includes Prague 4 with the highest number of persons over 60. We presume that for the first group one specialized workplace will be sufficient, for the second one or two workplaces and for Prague 4 more than two specialized workplaces – preferably decentralized ones. To get an idea about how busy individual Prague dis-

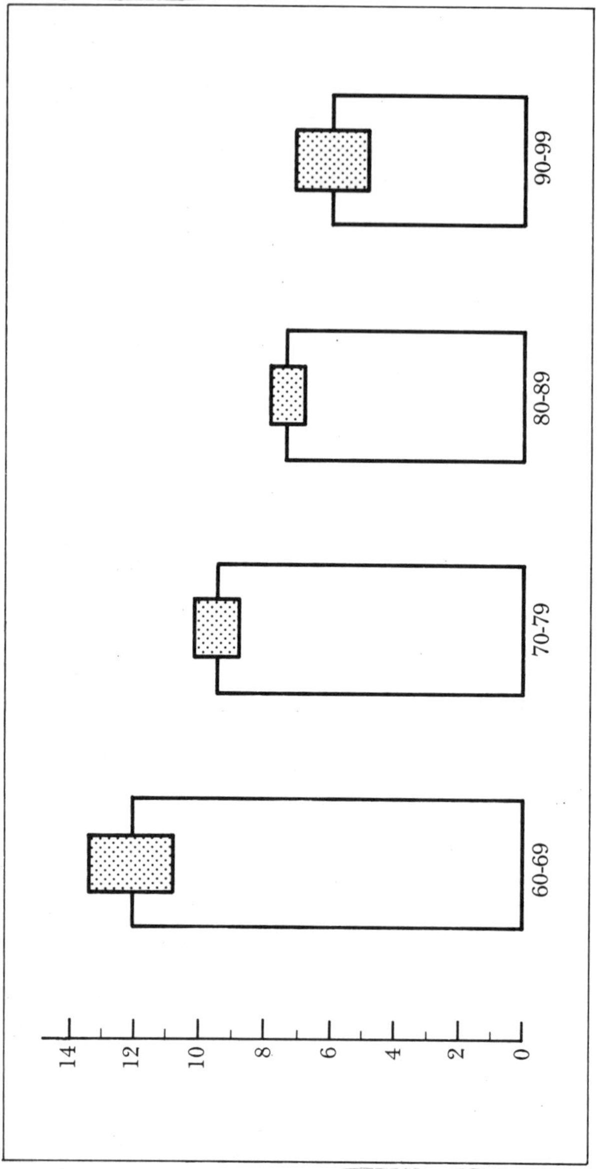

Fig. 9-3 Mean number of teeth for persons with natural teeth in different age groups.

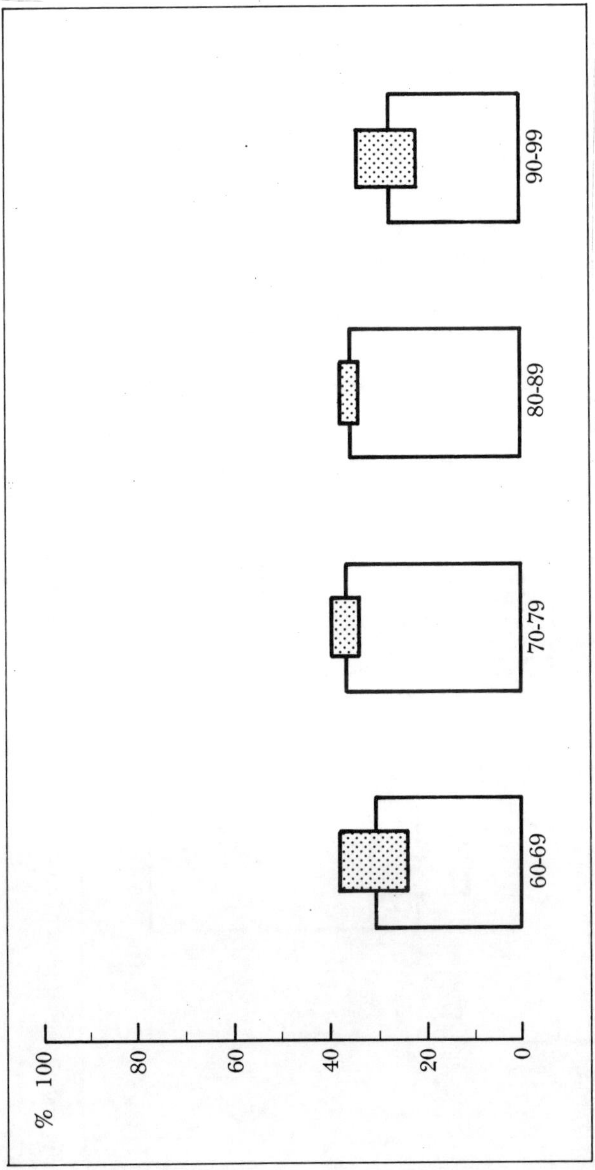

Fig. 9-4 Percentage of persons in nursing homes who utilized dental services in 1986.

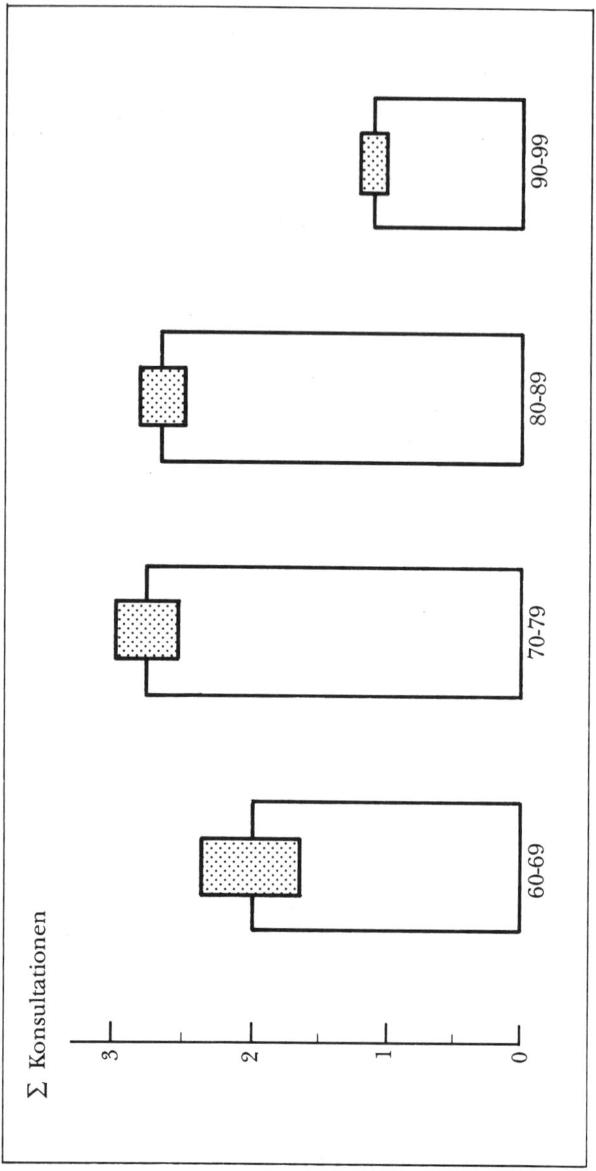

Fig. 9-5 Number of dental visits 1986 in different age groups.

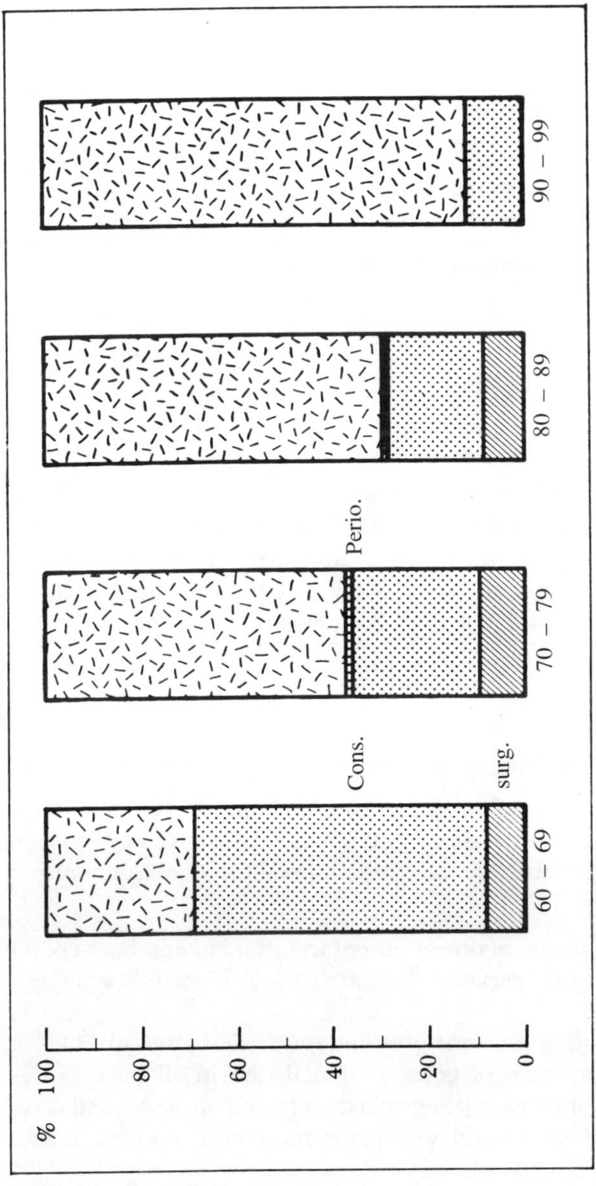

Fig. 9-6 Distribution of conservative, periodontal and surgical treatment in different age groups.

Table 9-2 Age grouping of persons over 60 in Prague districts

District	Number of inhabitants	Persons over 60	Age Groups 60-69	70-79	80-89	90-
Prague 1	47,163	8,240	3,930	3,082	989	239
Prague 2	66,938	11,700	5,581	4,376	1,404	339
Prague 3	86,807	15,190	7,250	5,775	1,824	440
Prague 4	289,019	50,570	24,130	18,915	6,065	1,450
Prague 5	106,504	18,630	8,872	6,973	2,243	524
Prague 6	137,124	23,990	11,448	8,972	2,880	690
Prague 7	51,628	9,030	4,298	3,385	1,085	262
Prague 8	124,017	21,700	10,350	8,115	2,606	628
Prague 9	122,714	21,470	10,250	8,030	2,572	617
Prague 10	162,959	28,500	13,627	10,640	3,410	823

tricts in geriatric dentistry are, we assessed the number of persons over 65 years per physician. We intentionally left out the age group of 60 to 64 because their treatment is not very different from that of middle-aged persons. At present in the area of Prague there are 280 persons over 65 per doctor.

Conclusions

On the basis of our previous experience and epidemiological investigation we recommend the following steps concerning geriatric dental care in medical establishments in Prague.

1. Setting up of one or more (according to number of older persons) geriatric dentistry centres in each Prague district.
2. Leading physician working there will be responsible for supervision of geriatric dental care in all districts. He should have a postgraduate diploma of the second class. The specialized workplace must have enough nurses

because of the exacting treatment, and laboratory technicians because of the predominance of dental prosthetic treatment.

3. To prepare, according to resources, dental workplaces in geriatric establishments. This will increase accessibility and the possibility of prevention.
4. Close cooperation between dentists and gerontologists in each Prague district, especially in prevention and treatment.
5. To include gerontology and geriatric dentistry, with emphasis on psychology and ethical aspects of pre- and postgraduate education.

We know that all the above-mentioned tasks cannot be implemented to such a wide extent, except in big cities where medical care is concentrated.

Bibliography

1. *Thomas-Weintraub, A.*
Dental needs and dental service use patterns of an elderly edentulous population. J Prosthet Dent 54: 526-532, 1985.

2. *Mani, N.J.*
Preliminary report on prevalence of oral cancer and precancerous lesions among dental patients in Saudi Arabia. Community Dent Oral Epidemiol 13: 247-248, 1985.

3. *Mazur, Z.*
Geriatric patient at stomatologist. Practical Stomatologist 36: 5: 150-158, 1987.

4. *Barmes, D.E.*
How to bridge the gap. Proceedings of the ADEE 1983 (Association for Dental Education in Europe).

Chapter 10
Problems and Perspectives in Geriatric Dentistry in the Soviet Union

N.N. Baschanow

The Soviet Union, like other nations of the world, has experienced a continuous increase in the proportion of the elderly and aged in its population. Such aging of the population leads to ever increasing percentages of elderly and aged patients in polyclinics and hospitals. In 1970, the elderly comprised 11.8% of such patients (more than 28 million persons); in 1975, the proportion had already increased to 13.2% (more than 30 million persons). A not insignificant proportion of this population group requires inpatient care.

Age-related and functional changes in all orofacial organs and tissues occur in the elderly. Among the oral changes tooth loss, followed by disturbances of function, is most frequent. According to *Bernadskij* et al. [1], 636 of 1000 subjects examined are completely edentulous in one or both jaws. That means that approximately 20 million persons require prosthetic treatment; *Rybakow* and *Basijan* [8] claim the number to be 28 million. Also notable for their frequency are atrophy of the jaw and alterations of the oral mucosa. The epidemiological pattern is dominated by marginal diseases, functional disturbances of the salivary glands, temporomandibular joint disease, odontogenic inflammation of the soft tissue of the face and neck and oncological disease.

Outpatient surgical intervention as a consequence of odontogenic inflammation is required in 54.3% of elderly patients [6] and 5% to 6.4% (several million patients) require hospitalization.
The complicating factor in the dental treatment of elderly and aged patients is the existence, in nearly all such persons, of one or more systemic diseases [8]. Thus, for example, 302 of 1000 subjects have one systemic disease, 40% have two, and 30% have five or more [7]. As a result, consultations and intervention by specialists in internal medicine and other disciplines are necessary in addition to dental therapy. Oral rehabilitation is required by 52.5% – more than 15 million persons [4].
Oral and maxillofacial surgical treatment of elderly and aged patients is frequently accompanied by complicatins, so that special nursing care is needed in addition to the basic therapy. Fifty per cent of patients over age 60 years require constant monitoring; 63% are completely unable to care for themselves [5].
Demographic investigations must include high-risk population groups as well. These include:

- very old persons (over age 90 years)
- elderly persons living alone (single person households without close relatives)
- severely ill elderly persons and those with mental retardation
- elderly couples, one of whom is physically or mentally disabled

At present, dental care for the elderly is organized as follows:

- organized care for specific population groups (assignment to specific polyclinics, care demand initiated by patients and through check-ups in dispensaries); this mode of care delivery is the most effective;
- war and industrial invalids who receive regular care, at home if necessary;
- hospitalized patients receive comprehensive dental care, including prosthodontic treatment;

- persons not included in such groups, who seek treatment as symptoms arise. This is the least effective form of care from the point of view of regular check-ups and maintenance.

At present, no single mandatory organization for dental care of the aged considers general medical and social factors in the Soviet Union.
A series of scientific studies dealing with geriatric dentistry has been made in the Soviet Union. The Kiev Medical Institute, directed by Professor *Bernadskij* [1], has considered the relationship betwenn loss of teeth and age, and with details of the clinical course and treatment of inflammatory processes in elderly patients. Similar goals motivated reports by *Grigontschuk* [3] and *Bugakow* [2].
Results of these studies, taken as a whole, indicate that many questions related to geriatric dentistry remain unanswered and that the entire subject requires further serious study. The need for exchange of experiences by experts in the socialist nations is a related aspect. It must be noted that the praesidium of the All-Union Scientific Society for Stomatology of the USSR has already discussed the problems of geriatric dentistry twice, and has developed a plan for the scientific solution of these problems through the dental schools of the USSR.
Epidemiological and public health studies must be directed toward specific problems, due attention being given to general medical and social factors. The first tactical task in optimizing dental care for the elderly is the formation of special care units in polyclinics and development of care collectives for dental home care delivery. Experiences reported in Leningrad regarding single day hospitalization for such patients are quite positive [6]. Long-term tasks may be classified as follows:

- studies of the epidemiological profile of oral diseases in the elderly and the aged;
- estimation of the type and character of care required;

- development of organizational principles for geriatric dental care;
- integration of geriatric dental care considerations into educational programmes in undergraduate, graduate and continuing education programmes.

Intensive cooperative efforts by dental researchers in the socialist nations will promote the rapid resolution of these important matters.

Bibliography

1. *Bernadskij, J.I.*
Entzündungen im Kiefer-Gesichtsbereich bei älteren und alten Patienten. Kiew »Gesundheit« 1987, S. 103.

2. *Bugakow, E.M.*
Klinik, Diagnostik und Therapie akuter Entzündungen im Kiefer-Gesichts- und Halsbereich bei älteren und alten Patienten. Autoreferat Md. Diss. 1987, S. 22.

3. *Grigortschuk, J.F.*
Klinik und Therapie von Phlegmonen und Abszessen des Kiefer-Gesichtsbereiches bei älteren und alten Menschen. Autoreferat Med. Diss. Kiew, 1987, S. 46.

4. *Jakowlewa, W.I., Kaminskij, A.M. and Bildjuschlewitsch, M.A.*
Stomatologische Erkrankungen bei Invaliden des zweiten Weltkrieges. Stomatol (Moskva) 4: 72-74, 1977.

5. *Kan, W.M.*
Analyse des Gesundheitszustandes bei über 60jährigen und einige Fragen zur medizinisch-sozialen Betreuung. pp 33-34 In: Probleme der theoretischen und klinischen Medizin in Entwicklungsländern M. 1975.

6. *Koslow, W.A.*
Dringende stationäre stomatologische Hilfe. Leningrad, M. 1988, S. 288.

7. *Rewuzkaja, S.G.*
Wege zur Entwiclung einer geriatrischen Betreuung. pp 108-112 In: Sozial-ökonomische Probleme der Gerostomatologie. Tbilisi, 1976.

8. *Rybakow, A.I. and Basigan, G.W.*
Epidemiologie stomatologischer Erkrankungen und Wege ihrer Prävention. M. M., 1973, S. 320.

Chapter 11
Fundamental Principles for the Development and Implementation of Geriatric Dental Care Programmes in the Republic of Bulgaria

Z. Jolov

The most reliable strategy for decreasing the gap between oral health care needs and their satisfaction, i.e. obtaining an acceptable oral health status, is the realization of the National Oral Health Programme, based on a preventive approach. In this way a large proportion of the oral health problems of the aged population will be solved.

Elderly people in the future will play a considerable role in the determiniation of oral health care needs, especially the needs of prosthetic care. The main factors influencing these needs are the following:

1. The unsatisfactory oral health status of adult and aged population groups at present.
2. The increasing life expectancy and percentage of elderly and old people.
3. The existing trend towards tooth lose in aged people because of periodontal disease, against which there are no effective preventive programmes.

Bearing in mind that nearly 17% of retired persons continue to work, that 27% are able to work and that 42% are able to work at light jobs, we considered that the social policy for special health care for aged people would have to include oral health care.

At the moment oral health care for elderly people is included in the general health care programme for adults. About 6500 elderly persons live in homes for the aged and receive regular oral health care. There are few studies considering the different oral health problems of the aged [1-4]. They indicate that serious oral health problems of the aged exist, and for their elimination special oral health care is necessary.

Because of the lack of comprehensive epidemiological data, a complete situation analysis of geriatric dental care is impossible at present, as is a national geriatric dental care programme.

Bearing in mind the significance of the problem, the number of dental personnel and the existing conditions of social care for the aged, we considered the development of a geriatric dental care programme with approximately the following structure:

Present condition and problems in dental care for the aged

1. Study of the condition and trends of health-demographic indices.
   The data for this will be taken from the National Statistics. Now in Bulgaria more than 17 % of the population is aged over 60. By the year 2000 this percentage will be nearly 18%, and 48% will be persons aged over 70.
2. Epidemiological study of the condition of the mouth and teeth. The method and recording of this will be unique and will be accepted of all countries participating in the study. This is the main problem in the situational analy-

sis, and will engage most of the participants in the development of the programme. The data we have at the moment are very scarce and the conclusions made from them will be unreliable. Some studies indicate that in the age group 60 to 77 years tooth loss through simple and complicated caries is 40 % and at the age of 80 to 90 it is about 19% The percentage of tooth loss because of periodontal disease is 48% at age 60 to 70 and 69,2% at age 80 to 90.

3. The organization of oral health care in Bulgaria at present. This allows a large proportion of the oral health problems of the aged to be solved without creating special geriatric dental services. Such services will probably be created at homes for the aged. The elderly are not a priority group at the moment. Such priority oral care exists for other population groups (schoolchildren and children, pregnant women, recruiters).

The purpose of the programme

At this stage it is very difficult to determine measurable and real objectives. This will be possible only after completing the epidemiological study. The probable goals which we will have in view are as follows.

1. People to have at least 20 natural teeth at the age of 60. Probably this goal will be amended after study of the oral health status.
2. Each person to have a completely healthy oral cavity at retirement.
3. To emphasize the role of the elderly in their own dental health.
4. Preventive measures for delaying geriatric dental changes in the chewing and maxillofacial region.

Programme strategy

1. Classification of the morphological and functional changes in the maxillofacial region connected with aging, and development of preventive measures to delay the processes of aging.
2. Maximum preservation of natural teeth and preventive measures for preservation of residual teeth.
3. Prevention of the injuries and changes in TMJ and utilization of contemporary prosthetic methods of treatment.
4. Utilization of precise prosthetic methods of treatment, especially for the lower jaw.
5. Effective measures for early detection and treatment of preneoplasms in the mouth.
6. Dental health education for elderly persons, with special reference to oral hygiene.
7. Inclusion geriatric dentistry topics in the dental student's curriculum.

Implementation of the strategy objectives and monitoring

Management and assessment

It is predicted that the management and evaluation of the programme will be carried out by a group of specialists, helped by the Ministry of Health and the Bulgarian Dental Association.
The analysis and evaluation system will correspond to the recommendations of experts in geriatric dental care.

Bibliography

1. *Bojanow, R. and Rajkowa, E.:*
   Gerostomatologische, prothetische Untersuchungen älterer Bürger der Stadt Sofia. Stomatologija, Sofia 53: 1, 1971.
2. *Stiljanow, G. and Bojanow, B.:*
   Zahnlosigkeit der Bevölkerung und Zustand der prothetischen Versorgung in Bulgarien. Stomatologija, Sofija 35: 2, 1953.
3. *Stiljanow, G. and Bojanow, B.:*
   Widerspiegelung der sozialen Lage auf die Zahnlosigkeit der Bevölkerung in Bulgarien. Stomatologija, Sofija 36: 1, 1955.
4. *Stranski, D.*
   Langlebigkeit und Zähne. Stomatologija, Sofija 47: 6, 1965.
5. *WHO*
   Oral Health Surveys. Basic Methods, 3rd ed. Geneva, 1987.

Part IV Recommendations

Chapter 12 Possibilities for Implementation of Geriatric Dental Care from the Point of View of the State

V. Šicha

The state health care system, including the dental treatment of older and senior citizens, can provide the elderly with their needs on the basis of daily practice and according to the epidemiological studies carried out.

It is obvious that the dental care of old people at the local level must be adapted to the infrastructural conditions from the viewpoint of both geriatric dental treatment and the organization of dental care.

From the papers delivered it is clear that in the dental treatment of older and senior citizens health personnel must play an active role. This concerns not only professional and highly skilled treatment but particularly active case-finding, active screening organized care and of aged patients who need this care. As we have already heard, these problems are for many reasons complex, and on many occasions unachieveable for dentists. The dentist must cooperate in this activity with a team of other specialists dealing with these problems.

The active case-finding of old and senior citizens who need dental care is easier when these people live in old people's homes or are under long-term or permanent treatment in hospitals for old and chronically ill people. Dental care here is a part of their whole treatment. Dental treatment is, then, from the personnel and technical point of view, quite possible, provided that the old person is convinced of the necessity of such treatment. In this respect the dentist must cooperate closely with other specialists, particularly general practitioners, psychologists, nurses who are specially trained for work with old people and with others who are working in these institutes.

When old people live out of reach of the above-mentioned establishments for social and health care, i.e. when they live with their families or are alone, their dental treatment is rather more complex, not only from the viewpoint of case-finding but also from the viewpoint of realization.

It is necessary for the dentist to cooperate with those in the social health care system, with general practitioners and gerontological-geriatric nurses who regularly visit these old people and provide them with health treatment. In addition, it is often necessary to win the members of the old person's family over for cooperation. Without the active help of family members, the dental care and treatment of the elderly would often be impossible.

The dental care of old people, provided that no special diagnostic and therapeutic equipment is needed, because of the character of their disease can, in our experience, be provided by the local dentist. He has usually known these patients for some years, and he may also have treated their younger family members, which makes the whole treatment plan easier.

When the dental treatment of older and senior citizens because of its exacting character, requires a more complex diagnostic and therapeutic approach, the patient should be treated by a specially trained dentist and his nurse. This dentist, specially trained in the treatment of old persons, should work within the polyclinic system, especially in the departments of dental prosthetics and surgery.

If old patients, especially those who have some problems with their mobility and live rather far from the place of treatment, need dental treatment, some beds should be reserved for them in dental departments. We are convinced that the treatment of hospitalized dental patients is easier, quicker and more effective, particularly in those cases when no surgical intervention is necessary. The treatment of hospitalized patients also involves treatment in the field of prosthetics, possibly conservative dentistry, etc. When an old patient is hospitalized, it is possible to apply the correct use and treatment of the dentures, necessary hygiene, and so on. Of course, together with the possibility of hospitalization of so-called non-surgical dental patients it is also necessary, while planning the number of beds for dental departments, to take into account the proper education of dental personnel in basic, pregraduate programmes and also in further education.

We would estimate that for the conditions prevailing in Czechoslovakia, according to the amendments to the Programme for the Field of Stomatology and with regard to the above-mentioned facts, 5 beds per 100,000 citizens in dental departments are required.

From the social viewpoint, we think that any correctly indicated and medically supported dental treatment of old people should be free of charge, because as a rule socially disadvantaged individuals are concerned.

Bibliography

1. *Dohnal, K.*
Komplexni zdravotne sociálnipéce o osoby vyssiho veku (Komplexe Gesundheits- und Sozialfürsorge für Menschen höheren Alters). Zdrav pracovnice 37: 197-204, 1987.

2. *Donek, E. and Donková, M.*
Stáry a psychika (Alter und Psyche) Prakt lek 68: 49-51, 1988.

3. *Haluza, P.*
Sociálni péce o staré obcany po XVII. sjezdu KSC (Soziale Fürsorge für alte Menschen nach dem XVII. Parteitag der KSC). Zdrav pracovnice 37: 191-196, 1987.

4. *Haskovcová, H.*
Cile a postoje osetrujicich v geriatrii (Ziele und Stellung der Behandelnden in der Geriatrie). Zdrav pracovnice 37: 211-214, 1987.

5. *Jarolimek, J.*
Sociálni lékarstvi (Sozialmedizin). Prag: Avicenum-Verlag, 1987.

6. *Kondás, O. and Hermánek, S.*
Psychologie v liecebnej rehabilitácii (Psychologie in der medizinischen Rehabilitation.) Verlag Osvèta, Martin 1976.

7. *Krivohlavý, J.*
Sociálni komunikace se starymi lidmi (Soziale Kommunikation mit alten Menschen) Zdrav pracovnice 37: 215-221, 1987.

Chapter 13
Geriatric Dentistry Training, Specialization and Continuing Education Requirements in Professional School Faculties

A. Dapecí

Many studies have shown that the number of people over 65 and particularly those over 80 years of age will increase in advanced European countries until the year 2000. Dental care of the elderly may take various forms in each country, according to its development, economics and way of organizing health care. In Czechoslovakia physicians have been working in the local system. Health care of the elderly and of long-term patients has been secured both by territorial local physicians and local dentists in out-patient departments, and in geriatric care institutions and in hospitals for long-term patients and for the elderly homes. These institutes have their special physicians and nursing staff. The activity of out-patient departments is secured by geriatric nurses who also provide home nursing care. For example, in the South Moravia Region, there are 296 geriatric nurses, approximately one nurse for two to three districts. Dental therapy for citizens over 60 years of age has not yet been secured as regards organization, and it is usually carried out by a district dentist [1].

An indispensable part of building high-quality dental care for the elderly is the education of specially trained experts who will have sufficient theoretical knowledge not only about dentistry but also about the diseases of old age, psychology of the elderly, and, particularly, about aspects of geriatric care generally. The teaching will have to cover all degrees of education, i.e. pregraduate and postgraduate training of both secondary and university staff [3]. The present situation of including geriatric dentistry in the training of health service workers differs in COMECON countries as well as in other states. As regards European countries, Denmark has very well organized education in geriatric dentistry. In the Danish universities gerontology is taught in 48 lessons, and this number should be increased to 150 to 200 lessons. The forms of teaching include lectures, seminars, affiliations, etc. In Denmark there are also dentists who specialize in geriatric dentistry. This specialization, however, is only possible because of the great number of dentists in Denmark; the dentist: patient ratio is 1:850. The inclusion of geriatric dental training is still sporadic in the pregraduate period, but it has become a part of postgraduate education in a number of countries, such as in the Netherlands, FRG and England [2, 4].

In medical faculties in Czechoslovakia geriatric dentistry has been included in the theoretical as well as practical education of dentists, not as a separate subject but as a component of education in individual dental disciplines. Geriatric dentistry is taught by a dental centre at the Institute for Further Education of Physicians in Brno in the postgraduate education of nursing and medical staff.

It has been shown that appropriate education of staff is indispensable for the development of geriatric dentistry and it should be organized in the course of pregraduate education in both the secondary schools of hygiene and in universities. Education which includes geriatric dentistry should become a part of post-graduate training. There should be also be relations with the education of specialized geriatric dental staff, graduates of general medicine and nurses acting as the initial contact with the elderly and getting to hear of their dental problems. If knowledge about geriatric dentistry increases systematically, it is possible to suppose that it will penetrate even into the sphere of prevention, hygiene and health education. We should assess whether making geriatric dentistry an independent branch, with relevant specialists acting within regions or other organizational units according to the situation in each country, would be appropriate.

Bibliograpy

1. *Jedlicka, V.*
Praktická geriatrie (Practical geriatrics) Brno, Ústav pro dalši vzdělávání středních zdravotnických pracovníku. 1984.

2. *Kinsey, J.G.*
A comparison of attitudes to geriatric dentistry in five EEC countries. Br Dent J. 161; 303-305, 1986.

3. *Martinson, I.*
Gerodontology comes of age. J. Gerodontol Nursing 10; 8-11 and 14-17, 1986.

4. *Watanabe I.*
Dental care of the elderly. Dentistry in Japan. Tokyo 1987, pp. 159-162.

Chapter 14
Recommendations
for "Further Development of Dental Care of the Elderly" in East European Nations

1. Introduction

This *recommendation* was adopted at the symposium on Geriatric Dentistry attended by experts from the Stomatology Associations of Socialist Countries and held in Brno (Czechoslovak Socialist Republic) on 25 and 26 May 1988. It is based on analyses of the epidemiological, demographic and health care situations in the various socialist countries and takes account of differences both in prevailing conditions and in scientific requirements. The recommendation will further the health policy goals set out in the communiqué issued by the Tenth Conference of Presidents and General Secretaries of the Stomatology Associations of Socialist Countries (Erfurt, German Democratic Republic, 1986). These goals are derived from the following international trends:

- An increase in the number of elderly people (over 65 years of age) with extensive tooth destruction and in need of dental care;
- The growing importance of geriatric oral health care in the socialist countries;
- The development of geriatric dentistry on the basis of re-

search-endorsed concepts covering both the psychosocial field and specific dental matters;
- Organizationally bringing the care offered into line with old people's physical and mental abilities to make use of geriatric dental services;
- The increasing integration of aspects of geriatric dentistry in training, further training and continuing education dispensed by dental schools and colleges.

The proposals set out in the *Recommendations* in the further development of dental care for the elderly are an expression of the common responsibility for health policy shared by the representatives of this speciality in the socialist countries and are designed to serve as scientific guidance for health ministries in practical implementation.

2. Situation assessment

Dental care is acknowledged as having reached a high level of quality in the socialist countries. In general, it may therefore be assumed that institutions providing dental treatment are available throughout each country and that access to them is guaranteed. Well-trained and highly qualified graduates of dental schools and colleges ensure qualitatively satisfactory dental care that is accepted by the population.

Laws and ministerial orders govern the systematic provision of dental care for women in pregnancy and early motherhood, for children and for the young people, as well as for a not inconsiderable proportion of the adult working population through institutions run by the occupational health services. Organized preventive dental care is increasingly beginning to be implemented, and the resulting improvement in the oral health status of the younger generation is becoming epidemiologically apparent in many places. It is increasingly clear that the question of dental care for defined population groups has been resolved or can be resolved within the foreseeable future. Thus it will be possible, and in part also necessary, to focus the efforts of dental care personnel on new areas of emphasis.

The oral health status and degree of dental care coverage of the elderly and old in individual countries are not always satisfactory. Unlike the systematic dental care provided for children and young people, comprehensively organized age-specific care for the elderly has so far been lacking.

In accordance with the strategic orientation of both the World Health Organization (WHO) and the International Dental Federation (FDI) – "Health for all by the year 2000 – Health through oral health" – global indicators for oral health by the year 2000 are to be applied in practice following their adaptation to national epidemiological conditions. For the socialist countries this involves the central task of ensuring that the benefits of socialist health and social policy are felt on the oral health of the elderly.

Theoretical and practical analysis of preventive oral health care, the phased implementation of comprehensive preventive care programmes and analysis of the dental care situation with regard to adults and the elderly have all clearly shown that oral health care primarily aimed at effecting a cure or rehabilitation must be reoriented towards *lifelong preventive care.* Satisfactory dental care of the population, in the sense of maintaining dental function right into old age, can become a reality only if such a strategy is put into effect, and this implies redefining the content of dental care. Crucial importance is attached to establishing organizational forms appropriate to the elderly with reference to:

- present and future demographic conditions;
- geographical analysis of the prevalence of oral diseases and the degree of dental care in age groups from 55 years;
- a more extensive understanding of the particular mental, physical and social conditions of the elderly and of their attitudes towards making use of oral health care services.

2.1 Demographic situation

Since the turn of the century the proportion of the world's population made up of the elderly has tripled, and this revolution in longevity is a process that will continue unabated. More and more people are living longer, and by the year 2000 the number of people over 60 is expected to have doubled.
Population aging is occuring in a particularly striking way in Europe. By 2000 the proportion of people over 60 will rise, in 19 out of 28 countries, from just over 18% to 22%, and in 2025 every seventh person is expected to be over 60 years old. Proportionately speaking, the expanding age groups in the population structure are thus those with quite extensive or extensive social/medical care needs, an observation which without doubt is also of relevance to strategies for the delivery of oral health care. As an expression of the higher life expectancy in the socialist countries, an increase in the proportion of people over 70 years old, in particular, is to be expected.
This demographic trend gives rise to the demand that demographic data must be obtained on the present and future age structure of the populations of all countries, in order to plan geriatric oral health care.

2.2 Epidemiological situation

While there is extensive information available on the prevalence of caries and gingivitis in young people, knowledge of the prevalence of oral diseases among the elderly and the degree of dental care required is limited.
International epidemiological comparisons show, however, that destruction of teeth due to caries or periodontal diseases does not become widespread until after the age of 55 years. It is estimated that people between 35 and 44 years old still have, on average, 24 natural teeth, but that figure falls steadily with age as a result of the appearance of sequelae to caries, progressive periodontal diseases and unnecessary ex-

tractions. At the same time, the proportion of people with no natural teeth to rises from some 1% in those between 35 and 44 years to 30% to 50% among those over 65. Expenditure on prosthetic treatment is considerable and requires an extensive input of dental care resources.
The oral health problems of the elderly are in addition made more acute by a number of physiological and pathological changes:

- atrophy of the oral mucosa and maxillofacial muscles;
- reduced salivation and a tendency towards xerostomia (as a result of taking medicaments);
- reduced sense of taste;
- pain on mastication with abraded teeth and those loosened by periodontal disease;
- frequent occurrence of prosthetics-related oral pathologies and oral infections (e.g. candidiasis, *Anguli infectiosi*);
- temporamandibular joint pain/disfunction syndrome;
- oral precancers (leukoplakia, lichen *planus*, etc.) and cancers of the lip and oral mucous membrane.

It should also be borne in mind that the vast majority of the elderly are faced with general health problems (infirmity, chronic diseases, mental changes) which themselves have an adverse effect on oral health status and uptake of dental care. Both oral health status and dental care coverage are accordingly worse among the elderly in need of care than in those who are physically fit and mentally alert.
From the dentist's point of view it should be emphasized that the quality of prosthetic treatment does not always meet the professional/scientific requirements laid down and that dentures are frequently worn for too long periods.
One essential prerequisite for planning geriatric oral health care is to carry out internationally agreed national epidemiological investigations to determine the present oral health status of the elderly and the resulting need for care. In this connection, information is required not only on the individual agegroups (55 to 64, 65 to 74, 75 and above), but

also broken down within these groups into those with full mobility and those in need of care in an institution or the family.

3. Geriatric oral health care – aims and activities

The change in the prevalence of oral diseases and loss of teeth clearly apparent in a number of countries justifies the recommendation to the effect that organized children's oral health protection, dental treatment and after-care (dental care for school children and adolescents) must be matched by a system of geriatric oral health care. The decision in principle to adopt such a long-term policy of health protection is dependent firstly on an effective dental care system being available and secondly on a genuine expansion – fully documented in demographic and epidemiological terms – of the need for dental care experienced by the elderly in a country. In order to meet the goal of improving both oral health status and dental care coverage in the different agegroups in a population, planning is required on the basis of pre-established health indicators. These include dental caries, the number of "natural" teeth still funtional and, as a final outcome of the oral disease process, "edentulousness" (International Dental Federation, 1982). Long-term dental care policies should thus be aligned on national oral health indicators, which in turn should be derived epidemiologically by comparison with the global indicators formulated. For the elderly, the latter are related primarily to retention of natural teeth and delimitation of edentulousness:

	FDI global indicators	*GDR national indicators*
Target 1	50% of children aged 5 to 6 years caries free	60% of children aged 5 to 6 years caries free
Target 2	No more than 3 DMF teeth at 12 years	No more than 3 DMF teeth at 12 years

Target 3	Full set of teeth in 80% of those aged 18 years	Full set of teeth in 90% of those aged 18 years
Target 4	50% reduction in edentulousness in the age group 35 to 44 years	24 natural teeth still functioning in the age group 35 to 44 years
Target 5	25% reduction in edentulousness in the age group over 64 years	50% of those over 64 years with 20 natural teeth, and nòt more than 25% edentulous.

These epidemiologically derived national oral health targets are to be attained by means of balanced programmes of dental care, to be implemented in defined phases up to and beyond the year 2000. The age group 35 to 44 years should therefore be seen as a particular target group: as a result of well-directed preventive measures over the next 15 to 20 years, they will reach the threshold of old age in a better state of oral health.
In the context of the concepts being given preference at national level, the preventive care and treatment dispensed to the elderly will, in the field of geriatric oral health, concentrate on the following tasks:

- Comprehensive rehabilitation of the mouth with the aim of preserving remaining teeth, restoring and protecting from abrasion the physiological jaw function, and preserving the denture bearing area. In this connection patients are to be enrolled in a programme of oral hygiene, preventive health care and treatment, in order to raise their health consciousness and their ability to maintain personal oral hygiene;
- High-risk patients from the dental point of view and those with physical, mental or social disabilities should be placed under a special individual care regime;
- In addition, the principles and specific forms of prevention-oriented treatment appropriate to each age group must be further developed on a scientific basis, and the organizational prerequisites for applying those principles in practical care must be met.

Particular attention should be paid to interdisciplinary cooperation in dentistry with geriatric psychology, psychiatry and sociology.

4. Organizational concept of geriatric oral health care

Geriatric oral health care should be developed as an integral component of the social and medical care of the elderly. In this respect both general and specific requirements should be imposed on its development, for which collective and individual aspects are respectively to be taken as a basis.
The organization of geriatric oral health care at regional level in a country should be aligned on the condition of the infrastructure and the physical ability of the elderly to make use of the dental care provided. To that end models of oral health care delivery both to those in old people's and nursing institutions and to those at home, should be drawn up and given phased implementation in practical care. In the present state of knowledge and in the light of practical experience, the following care models are to be recommended:

1. Establishment of special geriatric oral health consultation hours in central polyclinics and larger outpatient units, in which specialist care can be properly dispensed to elderly people "able to attend". These geriatric oral health centres should be given responsibility for regularly monitoring the oral health status of the elderly (at least once a year) and for carrying out treatment if required, as well as for oral hygiene measures given by qualified technical personnel under "call-and-recall" system.
2. In agreement with and with the support of family members, a system of preventive care and treatment should be developed to ensure that the necessary geria-

tric oral health care is given at home to elderly people who are physically disabled or in need of nursing care and who live alone or with their families. Regional dental care establishments should be made responsible for this. Co-operation between the geriatrician and the dentist, as well as between the dental nurse and the social worker (and/or community nurse), should be regarded as a basic prerequisite for accurately targeted and effective care of this high-risk group.

3. A similar system of preventive oral health care and treatment must also be developed for those living in smaller old people's homes and nursing homes, and at the least for the institutionalized proportion of those "unable to attend" a consultation, and for the elderly who are bedridden at home.
4. In order to provide regular geriatric oral health care to old people living in large old people's homes and nursing homes (e.g. with upwards of 300 people in need of care), it is recommended that "dental ambulances" should be introduced, equipped with the apparatus and instruments required to enable qualified dentists to give the necessary geriatric oral health care in the nursing setting (at the bedside) during set consulting hours; this should be done in close cooperation with the nursing personnel.

5. Qualification requirements for graduates of dental schools and colleges

The development of geriatric oral health care not only calls for policy decisions and better material conditions, it also imposes new and stricter requirements on the qualifications of graduates of dental schools and colleges.

Dental care of the elderly must be an integral part of basic oral health care; it thus does not call for specialization in the sense of specialist dental practitioners. However, the dentist active in the field of geriatric dentistry must have extensive knowledge of biology, psychology, nosology, physiology, geriatrics and sociology, and he/she must be deliberately trained to that end during his/her period of study and qualification as a specialist dental practitioner. So far as undergraduate training is concerned, dental schools are recommended to:

- include elements of geriatric dentistry in the disciplines of dentistry and medicine/psychology;
- hold practical clinical training sessions and require students in their clinical semester to carry out geriatric oral health care tasks in old people's homes and nursing homes.

The most effective and proper form of training must, however, be the creation of a complex multidisciplinary subject area of "geriatric stomatology", in which chairs can later be established.

Elements of geriatric dentistry imparting both an understanding of the scientific/theoretical foundations and practical skills should from now on be incorporated in the postgraduate training of dentists (stomatologists) and district general practitioners. Qualified and experienced dentists should be made aware, by means of furhter in-service training, of the particular tasks involved in geriatric oral health care, since it is to them that the job of breaking new ground in the development of geriatric oral health care must be entrusted.

Particular attention must be paid to the qualifications of graduates of dental technical colleges, since they will have a key role to play in providing care for the elderly. Similarly, medical nursing staff should be introduced to geriatric oral health problems, since the goal that has been set, namely to improve dental care for the elderly, cannot be attained without their cooperation.

Subjekt Index